LOVE YOURSELF LIKE A MAN

Self-Love For Men | How Being Vulnerable Is A Strength, Not A Weakness

REBECCA COLLINS

DISCLAIMER

The content contained within this book may not be reproduced, duplicated or transmitted without direct written permission from the author or the publisher.

Under no circumstances will any blame or legal responsibility be held against the publisher, or author, for any damages, reparation, or monetary loss due to the information contained within this book. Either directly or indirectly. You are responsible for your own choices, actions, and results.

Legal Notice:

This book is copyright protected. This book is only for personal use. You cannot amend, distribute, sell, use, quote or paraphrase any part, or the content within this book, without the consent of the author or publisher.

Disclaimer Notice:

Please note the information contained within this document is for educational and entertainment purposes only. All effort has been executed to present accurate, up-to-date, and reliable, complete information. No warranties of any kind are declared or implied. Readers acknowledge that the author is not engaging in the rendering of legal, financial, medical or professional advice. The content within this book has been derived from various sources. Please consult a licensed professional before attempting any techniques outlined in this book.

By reading this document, the reader agrees that under no circumstances is the author responsible for any losses, direct or indirect, which are incurred as a result of the use of the information contained within this document, including, but not limited to, — errors, omissions, or inaccuracies.

Copyright Rebecca Collins 2022 - All rights reserved.

10 WEEKLY NEWSLETTERS - FREE

FREE

10 **Weekly Issues of Rebecca's life-changing newsletter "Reclaim Your Power"** Rebecca covers Self Love, Self Esteem, Making Friends, Getting Your Life Back & Living A Life of Freedom.

https://rebecca.subscribemenow.com/

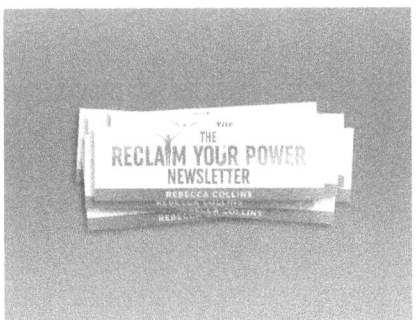

Scan with your smartphone's camera

CONTENTS

Introduction	ix
1. Self Love? But I'm A Man!	1
2. From Boys To Men	18
3. Big Boys DO Cry	30
4. Men Who Hurt Others Are Often Hurt Themselves	41
5. Say Goodbye To Low Self-Esteem For Good	53
6. The 7 Top Turn Ons In Men	67
7. Are You Helping or Hurting Others?	81
8. It's Time To Put It All Into Practice	90
9. A Love Letter To Yourself	99
Afterword	107
Sources	111
Notes	115

INTRODUCTION

- *"If you have the ability to love, love yourself first."* —Charles Bukowski

I grew up in a boy's world, being the only girl amongst four brothers. After hanging around with them so much, I often found myself having to behave like a boy just to fit in. Sometimes, that meant pretending to be tougher than I actually was. From falling off homemade go-karts while whizzing down the street at top speed to getting into punch-ups at 'friendly' football games, my brothers were resilient.

They never seemed to feel pain or show any emotions when they were sad. Wanting to be part of the gang back then, I learned all about this code of conduct for boys, which probably hasn't changed that much up to today.

Rule number one of the code was **never to cry** – not even when you had a bloodied nose or a banged-up knee after falling out of a tree. Number two was **never to get emotional**. Sure, you could get loud and angry, but being visibly upset was not what boys did. And, thirdly, **you had to be strong,** both physically and mentally if you wanted to be accepted and respected by the other boys.

I observed this unspoken code everywhere I went while growing up, from my school years and beyond. I watched as those boys became men, still staying true to the invisible code of how 'real men' should be.

It's usually society that conditions how we grow up, along with parental influences and cultural norms. It's almost impossible not to follow that template or behave in any other way when young. As we get older and develop a mind of our own, we might have different ideas about life or what it means to be a parent or partner, but some aspects of our upbringing stay with us.

One of those aspects is what it means to be a man (or woman) and there is a lot of pressure from outside to live up to that.

As a man, you are expected to behave in a certain way and exhibit specific attributes, just as women are expected to. When you think of all the things you are 'supposed' to be, a few adjectives probably come to mind, such as: strong, confident, brave, protective, and also be a rock to lean on. These are all wonderful qualities to have, right?

And then, there are the things you are NOT supposed to be: weak, insecure, afraid, sensitive, incapable. Of course, not all men are super confident or mentally strong. Most have insecurities and are extremely sensitive, but it isn't easy for them to show that when they are supposed to behave otherwise.

Although being 'macho' is now an outdated concept (thank goodness), many men feel confused about what being 'manly' actually means. On the one hand, they hear it is OK to be sensitive and caring and, on the other, feel like they won't be respected if they act too soft. Being a man is harder today than it has ever been and feelings of negativity and despair can creep in very easily. When you lose that sense of who you are meant to be, it can be devastating.

How do you navigate relationships, family, work, and life in general when society tells you, you are supposed to be invincible? If your emotions are always on lockdown, how do you take care of your mental health and self-esteem? For many men, self-love seems to be an overwhelming challenge and they just don't know where to start.

I'm glad you picked up this book, I've helped many men and women see themselves for who they really are. A beautiful soul and a wonderful person.

In my work as a life coach and mentor, I help men and women to feel more empowered and succeed in their life goals. Gender inequality still exists, unfortunately, so I have dedicated myself to enabling everyone to break through the stereotypes that history has placed on women.

But the same holds true for men and over the past few years, it has become obvious that many of them are also struggling. I recently began holding workshops for men who wanted advice on setting up their own business and after talking to them, one thing became very clear: **men are having a tough time trying to be tough all the time**.

While feminism gave a voice to women, many men feel voiceless and have lost sense of what their role is in life. If you are in your twenties or thirties, you might be finding it very hard to deal with the pressures of relationships in the dating culture. Social media has also created superficial ideas of what success looks like, causing a lot of young men to feel insecure about their appearance or capabilities.

If you are in your forties or fifties, you may still believe you have to be a certain kind of role model to your children or partner, and have a successful career. It's possible that you haven't been able to achieve any of these and now you feel like a total failure.

Men's mental health has recently become a talking point, with the focus turning to why so many men are suffering from depression and feelings of social isolation. It is frightening if you consider that the number of suicides among men is soaring. According to a report by the Mental Health Foundation UK[1] released in 2021, men's mental health is taking some battering. The figures speak for themself:

- Three times as many men as women die by suicide
- Men aged 40 to 49 have the highest suicide rates in the UK
- Men report lower levels of life satisfaction than women, according to the UK Government's national well-being survey

- Men are less likely to seek therapy than women: only 36% of referrals to the National Health Service counselling therapies are for men

In addition to all of the above, men are much more likely than women to go missing, sleep rough, and become dependent on alcohol or engage in frequent drug use. The figures are similar in the US, with the American Psychological Association reporting in 2015 that the suicide rate among American men is about four times higher than among women.[2]

The truth is that men are finding it hard to love themselves.

I want to address that problem, which is why I have written this book.

Although there are many self-help books already out there for women (**Love Yourself Deeply** being my favorite as it was written by me :-), but, you won't find many for men on the bookshelves.

That is a shame, because men are suffering and often find it incredibly difficult to seek help. I sincerely hope this book will change that and be a helping hand to you, or any man, who is feeling lost, lonely, and lacking in self-love.

While you might have a knee-jerk reaction to the term 'self-love', stay with me. As you go through the book, you will get some valuable insights into why self-love is important – even for you! It isn't just something for women – we all need to practice self-love. It is not about having facials or binging on a tub of Ben and Jerry's either. But it has everything to do with your happiness and well-being.

Self-love should never be confused with arrogance, selfishness or ego – it is more to do with nurturing your inner needs, fortifying your self-worth, and feeling comfortable with who you are.

Throughout the chapters in this book, I will be sharing some practical guidelines to help you reclaim the fundamental right to love yourself deeply and begin living a fulfilling, balanced life.

- I'll be talking about how going through the process from boy to man may have conditioned you to be someone you are not. You will find useful tips to help you work toward greater self-awareness.
- Depending on how you grew up, you might still be carrying a lot of trauma around with you that is affecting your everyday life. This book will gently allow you to heal and free yourself from negative self-beliefs.
- If you are hurting inside, you are probably hurting those around you too. You will find a safe space here to process and eliminate those destructive emotions and behaviors.
- If you feel very low and have lost all confidence in yourself, you will discover strategies to reclaim your sense of self-worth and self-esteem.
- If you feel right now that you are at the bottom of a very dark pit you can't get out of, I am here to tell you that you can and I'll be giving you the tools you need to climb up into the light.
- If you have relationship burnout and are left feeling battered and bruised, you will learn how to process those intense emotions and restore your self-esteem.
- If you feel like a failure and can't seem to live up to other people's expectations, you will learn how to value your inner man and deflect the negativity of others.
- If you need a friend to support you as you begin the journey of nurturing your inner needs and learning how to embrace the wonderful man you are, this book is for you.

When you learn about the power of self-love, you will realize that being true to yourself is much more manly than trying to be someone else or putting on a brave face.

I believe that you can be whoever and however you want to be. I know that, as a man, you can be strong, confident, brave, and a real rock. I also know that you can be sensitive, nurturing, caring, and very loving.

It's time for you to liberate those precious qualities you have been keeping locked away for so long. If you can reach deep inside to find your authentic self, you will get to know an amazing person. He is your buddy, your best friend, your role model, and your confidante. He is the real man you have always been.

Once you begin taking care of yourself, you can also take care of others and begin to experience a truly wonderful life.

It all begins with self-love.

I
SELF LOVE? BUT I'M A MAN!

- *"The hardest challenge is to be yourself in a world where everyone is trying to make you be somebody else."* – E. E. Cummings

On a recent night out with a group of women friends, I noticed how naturally the conversation turned to the importance of taking some 'me time', self-pampering, and practicing self-care. From pedicures and spa days to girl-only weekends, women are seizing the opportunity to prioritize themselves even when they have demanding lives and countless responsibilities.

They recognize that self-love is crucial to their well-being and makes for more fulfilling relationships.

Afterwards, I realized just how easily it had become for women to express their needs while most men find that extremely difficult to do. In a society that still expects the male figure to be the breadwinner and able to cope with all of life's problems, most men don't practice self-love. Instead, they have learned to put their feelings and needs to one side, along with any signs of vulnerability or weakness.

The idea of self-love itself might sound like a girl thing to you – something that applies to women and not relevant to men like you. You could even be under the impression that there is some kind of sexual meaning behind it. Well, self-love is none of the above so let's find out what it really means and why you should begin to incorporate it into your life.

What is self-love?

Here are a few definitions of self-love:

- an appreciation of your own worth or virtue
- proper regard for and attention to your own happiness or well-being
- recognizing that your own needs and wishes are important

As you can see, it is all about looking after your well-being, but not in a selfish way. Inner happiness comes when you feel good about yourself as a person, not when you despise who you are. When you learn how to do that, everything changes. No matter what problems you are facing in life, having a solid belief in your worth and value means you can weather the storms without any collateral damage. Self-love is really the anchor to keep you safe, happy, and balanced.

Put it this way: the more you love yourself, the more love you will spread to others, and the more you will receive in return. That's what we all want at the end of the day, isn't it? To love and be loved?

Self-love begins with you and the relationship you have with yourself. Here are some questions you might never have asked yourself before. Think about each one and try to answer as truthfully as you can and see how well you treat and appreciate yourself. It is time to meet the man inside you. Are you ready? Let's go then.

Choose from the answers a, b, or c, as you work through the questions. You can write the answers down if you are listening to this book on audio.

When you look in the mirror, do you

a) Hate what you see?

b) Feel indifferent?

c) Feel good about yourself?

Do you forgive yourself easily?

a) No, I can't.

b) I try, but it isn't always easy.

c) Yes. I try not to repeat my mistakes.

How often do you give yourself a pep talk?

a) I don't need to talk to myself.

b) I give myself pep talks sometimes.

c) Regularly. I am my greatest cheerleader.

Do you find it easy to say 'No' when asked to do things you would rather not do?

a) I have a really hard time saying no.

b) I do, but I usually feel bad about it afterwards.

c) Yes, I do.

What three compliments would you give yourself right now?

a) I will have to think about it.

b) I can only think of one.

c) Only three? Here goes…

Do you put your own needs first or put those of others first?

a) It would be selfish to put my own needs first.

b) Sometimes, but I feel very guilty when I do.

c) It depends on the situation.

Do you take time out to exercise, eat healthily and pamper yourself?

a) I don't have time for that.

b) Not as often as I would like to.

c) Sure. I work out regularly, watch what I eat, and enjoy my free time.

Do you accept yourself, even the parts you don't like?

a) I don't like anything about myself.

b) I try but sometimes it isn't that easy.

c) I accept how I am and can live with it.

Do you set and maintain boundaries with people?

a) I don't think you can have boundaries with people you love.

b) I try, but find it difficult to do it all the time.

c) Yes, I do because it's important for my well-being.

Do you have a support network of friends you can rely on when you need them?

a) I don't like confiding in people.

b) I think there are a few people I can confide in but I'm not too sure.

c) I have a great group of friends who are always there for me.

How often do you compare yourself to others?

a) All the time.

b) I try not to, although I find myself doing it a lot.

c) I can't see the point of that. Everyone is different.

Do you feel that you are a lovable person?

a) Not really...what's to love?

b) Sometimes, but I don't really think about it that much.

c) Sure. I am as loveable as the next man.

The questions above will hopefully give you some insight into how much self-love you are practicing or denying yourself.

If you answered mostly *a*, your discontentment about life could be coming from low self-esteem and a lack of self-value. It is also likely that you find it hard to express yourself and trust your own judgment. You may not know where all of that is coming from but you have made an important step in acknowledging that this could be the case. Throughout this new learning process, you can become the man you want to be.

If you answered mostly *b*, you probably struggle on some occasions to know how to act and have a tendency to ignore your emotions. This can make you feel dissatisfied and unhappy with your life, although you don't have the skills to figure out exactly where you are going wrong. Hopefully, you will gain a better understanding of how to reconnect with your inner needs in this book.

If you answered mostly *c*, you are likely to feel well-balanced and have a healthy dose of self-esteem. You respect your mind and body and embrace self-love as a way of life. If that is the case, I hope you can give this book to someone who needs it when you have finished or share the tips you have learned with your male peers. They might be struggling to handle their issues and you can offer them support and guidance.

Self-love means making friends with yourself

As funny as it may sound, if you don't like yourself, you can't expect others to like you. The more you down-talk yourself, ignore your needs, and abuse your emotional health, the more discontent you are going to feel. Is this how you would treat your friends? I am sure the answer is no because if you did, they would drop you in a split second.

Even though you might find it acceptable to kindly tell a mate not to worry when they are stressed out, or *"good job"* when they do something well, how often do you tell yourself the same things? When was the last time you said to yourself, *"I am so proud of you. I appreciate you. You did the best you could"*?

Self-doubt, self-criticism, and insults are harmful activities that eat away at you over time. You wouldn't expect your friends to treat you this way, vent their anger on you, or bully you, yet it's quite possible you have been doing that to yourself for a good while.

When this goes on long enough, it becomes your reality – a self-destructive habit. But habits can be broken. When you start treating yourself like a friend instead of being your own worst enemy, you will begin to feel differently. You will have greater trust in your abilities, feel more confident about who you are, and experience life through a completely new lens.

Self-love means love talk

You know that conversation happening in your head – the one that goes on and on about how useless, weak, or stupid you are? That's a learned thought pattern and you are so used to it that most of the time you don't even notice it's there. You might have been brought up to think that tough love works, but in this instance, all you are doing is punching yourself in the face every time you self-criticize.

Negative self-talk is very toxic and will never make you feel good about yourself. Imagine, for instance, Usain Bolt telling himself what a failure he was every time he lost a race (he did lose some – really).

He wouldn't have had the fortitude and positivity to go on and run the next race, and the one after that. Top athletes don't scold themselves when they miss a shot or lose a game – they put it behind them and carry on. There is no little voice in their head telling them how bad they are, only a positive one saying, "You've got this!"

The fancy word for negative self-talk is rumination – it's when you talk down to yourself constantly. This can eventually make you hate yourself and be full of self-loathing.

If it goes on for too long, it can be one of the factors that contribute to social anxiety, depression, and being unable to cope with even simple everyday events. Dwelling on all of your perceived negative traits also means that you never get around to addressing them or making any changes for the better.

Self-love means expressing emotions

Unfortunately, getting emotional isn't normally encouraged amongst males in society. That has traditionally been left to women to do, who are allowed to express how they feel. Men, on the other hand, are supposed to 'keep it together', no matter what they are going through.

There is nothing abnormal about showing emotions, although it could be that you just never learned how. Maybe you were always discouraged from showing your feelings and did not experience outward signs of affection while growing up.

Perhaps you work in a very male-dominated environment where the idea of being expressive would be misinterpreted or frowned upon. But here's the thing: we all need to express our emotions because we all have them.

Many men have bad experiences of showing their feelings or being emotional with women, getting called names like *pathetic, having no balls, a wimp*, and so on.

In reality, when you are in tune with your emotions and express them freely, you are practicing self-love. This leads to greater self-esteem and it won't matter to you if other people are not emotionally mature enough to understand where you are coming from.

Self-love means balance

You may be tempted to think that self-love is the same as smugness – the guy who brags about how he has it all and thinks he is better than everyone else. In reality, people like that probably have more insecurities than you can imagine. Thinking you are awesome is very different from thinking you are superior to others and putting yourself on a pedestal. No one likes a narcissist or an 'I'm in love with myself' kind of guy.

Self-love reflects neither of these traits. It's about recognizing who you are, where you come from, your strengths and weaknesses, and the progress you make toward becoming a better person. All of these come together to form a more balanced, loving, and understanding human being.

Self-love means self-respect

Women are encouraged more than ever today to focus on their inner strength, beauty, and power. Even though we still live in a male-dominated society, men are never told to seek their inner qualities but are expected instead to conform to some old-fashioned version of what it means to be masculine. As a result, many men become victims of the system they are part of, thinking they have to disrespect women, act aggressively, be 'hard', and be homophobic.

The only way to create a better world is if we all do it together and that means transcending old-fashioned gender roles and stereotypes. This book is written for anyone who feels they can relate to the problems it raises and is suffering from a lack of self-love, no matter what their sexual orientation is. At the same time, the issue of gender is too important to be mentioned briefly in one chapter and deserves a separate book of its own.

When you can develop a deep sense of self-respect for yourself, this has a ripple effect, extending to those around you. If you feel angry, stifled, and frustrated, this can lead to behavior that is disrespectful to others. You might then be consumed by guilt and self-loathing. If you can concentrate on developing self-respect for yourself, then you can share respect, empathy, and compassion for others.

Self-love means liberation

If you were deprived of love, understanding, support, and affection while growing up, you will find it difficult to share those qualities with others. You may have never learned how to love or were even given the impression that love hurts. Love never hurts when it is authentic, but people can hurt us. You are probably an expert at hurting yourself and this toxic relationship you have with your inner self can be very destructive.

When you experience self-love, love flows from you like a fountain. It is actually your inner strength and your secret weapon, liberating you from damaging fears and insecurities.

You might not have had the privilege of growing up feeling safe or loved, which is all the more reason why you have to begin embracing yourself now. When you love yourself, the world will love you back but the source of that love lies within you. You simply need to tap into it, nurture it and believe in it.

You can begin by trying to introduce some new habits into your life, starting now. Take a look at the points in the list below and choose three that you think you need more of in your life. Which ones are missing or are difficult for you to do? There is no pressure here to try to implement every point on the list from the word go. Simply think about your needs and how you would like to feel. With time, this new way of treating yourself will become a healthy habit that nourishes you from the inside out.

Let's take a look at what you can do to bring more self-love into your life:

- Talk about yourself with love (ignore the negative inner voice)
- Prioritize your needs (they are important)
- Avoid harmful self-judgment (no one is perfect so cut yourself some slack)
- Trust in yourself (you can do it!)
- Be honest with yourself (the truth is always better than a lie)
- Be nice to yourself (no guilt attached)
- Forgive yourself when you behave badly (learn from your mistakes and move on)
- Set healthy boundaries (maintain your space and don't let others use you)
- Indulge in your hobbies and interests (do what you enjoy)
- Take care of your health (both mental and physical)
- Do something creative (rediscover that playful young boy inside you)
- Treat yourself now and again (you deserve it!)

Self-love means accepting yourself as you are, including your emotions,, and looking after your physical, emotional, and mental well-being. When you can do that, you will feel more whole, happy, and content. You owe it to yourself to live life to the full and experience all the joy it has to offer you.

Self-love means self-care

While it's honorable to care for others and put your needs to one side, that can tip the balance the wrong way if you totally neglect your own needs. If you don't nourish your mind and body, how can you fully show up for someone else?

When you are on an airplane and the signal comes on to wear your oxygen mask, you have to put your own on first before you attend to your kids. This is the rule – save yourself first if you want to save others. It's not a selfish act but is more like common sense. You won't be of much use to anyone if you pass out and those around you who are vulnerable are left to fend for themselves.

This applies to everything you do: care for yourself so you can have enough energy to care for others. Men have traditionally been seen as the protectors but if they aren't protecting themselves, how can they protect their loved ones? When you give all the time without receiving, you will soon be running on empty and feel completely drained.

This is often called burnout and that's exactly what it is... fire needs oxygen to burn and if you starve it of that, you will self-extinguish!

The top 10 strategies to begin your journey of self-love

Your story is unique, which is why only you know what your needs are and what works for you. The good thing is that you can start practicing self-love with some very simple routines.

It doesn't have to be dramatic, or mean upending your whole life. It's more about the journey inside to rediscover who you are and what matters to you the most. I can honestly say that once you set off on this road to self-love, you will feel like a different person. The truth is that it will take you closer to the real you – the authentic you that has been struggling to find his way for so long.

Strategy 1: Create space to decompress

When you get up each morning, you might immediately start running around, seeing to the needs of your family or partner, rushing to work to start the daily grind, then getting home exhausted at night after a long day of obligations. You just don't have any time to yourself and even on the weekend, there are things you need to do – be that jobs around the house, helping out a buddy, or taking the kids to their various activities.

It can be really tiring and you do it because you are expected to. That's all fine, but you need to create some space for yourself in your daily schedule.

Why not set some time aside where you can do whatever you want to do? It can be anything from 10 minutes to an hour – depending on what is going on in your life. You don't have to plan anything special – it could be a walk around the park by yourself or a trip to the gym. When you make space, it gives you a chance to recharge. Apart from that, it is a positive step toward acknowledging that you have needs, too.

Even if you can't manage to do this every day, at least find a couple of days during the week when you spend time with yourself, guilt-free.

Strategy 2: Forget escapism and tune into creativity

It's easy enough to spend your free time zoning out with gaming but this is a bit like escaping from reality. I'm not saying don't enjoy a quick round of your favorite game, but when that is all you do, you are not creating anything. You are just killing time and numbing out emotions, thoughts, and feelings.

How about using your skills and imagination to make something from nothing? We humans are experts at that and there's nothing more satisfying than indulging in your creative passions.

If you don't feel you can be creative or have no idea where to start, just think about what you liked doing when you were a kid. Were you into skateboards, drawing, reading comic books, or climbing trees?

Whatever it was, you can start to rekindle those activities and get a real kick from making something from scratch. Why not create your own comic books, design skateboards, or build a treehouse? Doing whatever comes to you naturally, even if not perfect, will give you a great sense of achievement and accomplishment.

Strategy 3. Celebrate your small victories

Every day is a chance to celebrate your small victories. You do not need to wait for big things like a promotion or your team winning an important game to get excited. It will be a very boring life if that is the case, forcing us into a kind of zombie-like existence where we don't get fired up about anything anymore.

Think small instead, and give yourself a pat on the back whenever you get to work on time (yes, that is a victory for most people!), do something nice for someone else like making your mum a cup of tea, going to the gym three days in a row (that takes guts), and so on.

Whenever you do something well, you deserve to celebrate. What has this got to do with self-love? It means that you begin to start appreciating yourself and feel more positive about your capabilities. That's definitely something to celebrate!

Strategy 4. Get your day off to a positive start

Instead of waiting until the last minute to roll out of bed each morning, here is a great way to kickstart your day. Set your alarm to go off 30 minutes earlier than usual and do some stretching before 20 minutes of cardio.

You could go for a run or a cycle ride if you are up to it. After that, spend 10 minutes getting into a positive headspace with meditation or listening to a motivational podcast.

Avoid checking emails or your social media feed – these are stressors and you don't need them at this time of the day. Instead, make yourself a proper breakfast – not a coffee on the go – and enjoy it while reading a couple of pages from a book or writing down your goals for the day.

This routine can make all the difference to how you feel about yourself because you are feeding your sense of well-being and positivity. This is self-love 2.0 and even if you don't manage it every day, you will soon see what a difference it makes in your life and it can become a new habit!

Strategy 5. Maintain your boundaries

Relationships are built on give and take, but if you are doing all the giving, it's no wonder you end up feeling drained. Even if you love your family, friends, or partner, that doesn't mean you have to let them walk all over you.

Being a people-pleaser means you ignore your own needs and that can be self-destructive. Even though setting boundaries in your relationships may sound hard to do, they actually protect you from a lot of grief. As well as that, people then know where they stand with you and will be much less likely to try to take advantage of your good nature.

The way to set boundaries is to think of all the experiences that have made you feel uncomfortable or caused you pain, distress, and frustration. For example, saying yes every time your girlfriend wants you to go shopping with her may seem like no big deal. But if you don't really enjoy it and would prefer to spend your time doing something else alone or with your buddies, you need to set boundaries.

Having to change your plans at the last minute because a friend needs a lift somewhere is also an example of people overstepping the mark and you don't need to feel obliged to do anything that you don't want to.

If anyone is impacting your values and inner peace, you have to draw the line and make it clear you are not happy with that situation. The people who love and respect you will understand this, especially if you explain to them how you feel.

You might face negative reactions or accusations of being selfish but stand your ground – this kind of emotional manipulation is an unhealthy response. Lead by example and stay true to your values and levels of self-respect.

Strategy 6: Free your mind

I know that you might think meditation is a girly thing, or too woo-woo for you, but hear me out because you might have misunderstood what it is all about. Your mind is a powerfully efficient machine and it never stops working. Even when you are asleep, it's processing data, crunching numbers, and backing up information into its hard drive (or long-term memory).

On top of that, it is constantly trying to process experiences, put things into boxes, and tell you what to think. Neurons are firing off signals that help to create a circuit board you are plugged into 24/7, even if you are not aware of it.

Sensory overload can create stress and anxiety, sometimes causing that circuit board to blow a fuse and that's when you crash. To prevent this from happening, you can try some simple meditation – ten minutes a day at first is enough.

How can meditation help you? If you sit down, close your eyes, and allow your mind and body to relax, this has an extremely calming effect. As thoughts come and go, all you have to do is let them pass by, just like clouds floating past in the sky above you.

As you inhale and exhale slowly, you will begin to feel more grounded and at peace with yourself. Your problems will still be there afterward, but you will be in a much better position to face them with clarity and calmness.

Strategy 7. Make time for you

Everyone needs some time for themselves to do the things they enjoy. I can't emphasize enough how important it is for your well-being to create a few hours in the week to pursue your interests and hobbies. You do not need to make excuses to anyone about this or explain the justifications for it. You NEED to have time to yourself – end of story.

If people around you try to make you feel bad about this, remember that they are coming from a place that serves their best interests, not yours. Stay true to yourself and know that you deserve to indulge in some personal time if you want to feel good about yourself.

Strategy 8. Keep away from negative people

Very often, it's the people closest to us who bring us down. They might think they have a right to criticize us or remind us of our weaknesses every chance they get. Even friends can be a negative influence on us and often find it acceptable to tell us we will never get anywhere, do anything, or be anyone. When you are involved in any kind of toxic relationship, it can destroy your feelings of self-esteem and that is not what you need.

As difficult as it may be, you need to spend less time with these people and more time with those who will bolster your confidence, support your decisions, and have your back. While it might seem impossible to extract yourself from a close relationship with a family member such as with a sibling or parent, you can cut down the amount of time you spend with them to a minimum.

As for partners, friends, and other close connections, if they are bringing negativity into your life, you need to let them know that it isn't acceptable to you. If they don't change their attitude toward you, you need to move on.

Strategy 9. Seek intimate relationships with people who matter

The ones we love are often the ones who hurt us the most, unfortunately. That's because we have formed an intimate bond with them and made ourselves vulnerable. You might have been hurt in the past and decided never to get close to anyone ever again. I can understand why you would feel that way but there is nothing more fulfilling in life than sharing a deep, intimate bond with someone who truly loves and cares about you.

If you decide to be single because that just makes more sense to you, that is fine, too. A lot of people are, and you don't need to be constantly in a relationship. But what you can do is choose your next relationship carefully.

Think of what your needs are and your limitations. Consider what went wrong in the last relationship and work on getting it right this time. Establish ground rules from the start and set boundaries. Talk to your partner about your past experiences and listen to what they have to say, too.

Most importantly of all, allow yourself to be vulnerable because this is how love enters your heart.

Strategy 10. Fall in love with life

Remember those feelings of joy you had as a kid when playing with friends, watching a funny movie, and being downright silly? Being grown up doesn't mean that you have to stop having fun. In fact, all the more reason why you should!

While life might be very serious, with a load of responsibilities on your shoulders, you can still experience moments of unabashed joy and laughter. Everyone feels better when they have had a good laugh as they get a super boost of the feel-good hormone, serotonin.

Try to think about what you loved doing as a kid – what made you laugh and put you in a great mood? Even recalling those moments will put you in a positive mood now, helping you to go through each day with more positivity.

It is perfectly ok to laugh at yourself too, which is a sure sign of self-love. Instead of feeling stupid because you slipped on the banana skin, have a chuckle about it and laugh until your sides ache. There's no better feeling!

I think you can now see self-love is something that all men should experience. It strengthens you emotionally, mentally, and physically, making you feel more balanced and fulfilled.

Self-love really is your superpower and you are the hero of your story!

Highlights

- **Self-love means an appreciation of your worth, regard for your own happiness or well-being, and recognizing that your own needs are important.**
- **Establishing a healthy relationship with yourself is the key to happiness.**

- Being your own best friend instead of your worst enemy is a good starting point for practicing self-love.
- The negative voice inside your head is a bad habit that you can change into a positive one.
- It is normal to have feelings and expressing them reasonably is essential for your emotional well-being.
- Everything in life is about balance and when you can achieve that inside yourself, you can handle anything that comes your way.
- People around you may not respect you if you don't respect yourself first.
- When you begin to love yourself, you become free of all the negativity you have been carrying around with you for so long.
- Take care of yourself, then you will be in a better position to care for others
- Follow my top 10 strategies for self-love and enjoy life to the full.

2
FROM BOYS TO MEN

"If boys don't learn, men won't know." –Douglas Wilson

When Peter Pan first flew into Wendy's room in the famous children's story by J. M. Barrie, he told her he had run away from home the day he was born. When asked why, he replied that he never wanted to become a man. *"I want always to be a little boy and to have fun...."* he said. That's a wonderful dream and if only we could always stay young.

But everyone grows up, and the transition from boyhood to manhood is never an easy one. Maybe Peter Pan knew what he was talking about after all.

Raising boys

Back in reality, your idea of what it means to be a *real man* is shaped to a large extent by your experiences as a boy. From the day you are born, you will be treated differently than if you were a girl. It might not be anything obvious at first, and your parents or carers aren't necessarily doing it on purpose.

They probably will dress you in blue (because boys don't wear pink...) and will choose toys for you they think are 'boyish', like cars and trucks. They will even talk to you differently. Parents talk to their baby girls in a much more affectionate way than they do to boys.

A study from 2014 published in the journal Pediatrics[1] showed that mothers interact vocally more often with their infant daughters than they do with their sons.

Another study from Frontiers[2] revealed that mothers used more emotional words when talking to their 4-year-old daughters and were more likely to speak to them about emotional subjects. Fathers, too, were seen to use more emotional language with their 4-year-old daughters than with their 4-year-old sons. These subtle differences in communication do affect how boys eventually behave when they grow up.

In our culture, at least, we often send mixed messages to boys, so it's not surprising that they can get confused. One minute, we laugh off their behavior by saying, 'boys will be boys', and the next, we are telling them to 'grow up and act like a man'.

That's a very difficult expectation to live up to when you are just a kid. While it's the job of the parents or carers to guide boys into manhood to become strong, caring individuals, that doesn't always happen.

Especially by the time a boy has reached adolescence, his desire for independence can cause serious turmoil within the family and this is the age when many youngsters have their first run-ins with the law, start having trouble at school, show increased aggression, and begin experimenting with illegal substances or alcohol. The more conflict they experience with parents and teachers, the more they want to break free.

A lot of the time, adults have this idea that boys don't have feelings, thoughts, ambitions, or the ability to make their own decisions. Instead of nurturing these qualities in them, they demand that they follow their rules, their plans, and their view of the world. Rather than providing boys with options, they try to mold them into their idea of what it is to be a 'real man', just as their parents probably did to them.

As a girl, I know that I was treated differently from my brothers – not because my parents were bad. They simply didn't know any other way. I was protected more, especially as I reached my teen years, while my brothers were given a lot of free rein. If you can relate to this, you also need to know that it is never too late to break those patterns and become the person you want to be.

Perhaps your parents avoided kissing or hugging you because they thought it would make you soft. They probably discouraged you from crying too and expected you to swallow your feelings. This type of conditioning can have a lifelong effect on the way you view yourself and on what behavior you believe is allowed or unacceptable. I think you know what I am talking about.

Here are some labels that our culture (parents/teachers/society) tends to stick on boys. Of course, not everyone follows these stereotypes and there is a lot more being done today to counteract damaging ideas about what men (and women) are like. Having said that, some of the usual preconceptions still exist, as you can see below.

MEN ARE

Breadwinners

Violent

Aggressive

Mean

Bullies

Tough

Angry

Strong

Successful

In control

Leaders

Confident

Sexually active

Have no emotions

Can stand up for themselves

Can take it

Don't make mistakes

Don't cry

Take charge

Push people around

Know about sex

Don't back down

Take care of things

Can fix anything

Like fighting

Love sports

These are just some of the ways men are meant to be and behave. They are spoken and unspoken truths passed down from one generation to the next and if you don't fit in with these attributes, you are not viewed as a *real man*. That's a lot of pressure to be under, especially in your formative years. It's no wonder that many men feel stressed and under pressure to perform. In reality, a lot of men actually feel:

Confused
Angry
Scared
Stupid
Ashamed
Alone
Insecure

Powerless
Hopeless
Vulnerable
Worthless

Many parents will be shocked to know they raised boys who grew up feeling this way. They won't have realized that they are reinforcing these stereotypes of how boys 'should be'. If you were told to stand up for yourself when you were younger or encouraged to play sports, your parents were probably coming from a place of good intentions.

They would not have thought about the messages they were passing on to you or the values you were picking up from their advice.

It's likely that you were never told it is ok to express your feelings in words, or through art, music, writing, or dance. I can already hear you say, "Me? Dance? No way." Fair enough ... not everyone is going to be drawn to that kind of self-expression, and that's ok. But the point is, what if you had been encouraged to express your emotions in a safe, fun, supportive space?

What do boys need?

Boys are fully capable of being creative, caring, intelligent, and emotionally-balanced members of society if they are offered the opportunity. They can grow into loving, compassionate, healthy men if given half a chance.

I want you to think about what your needs are today. **These are the same needs you had when you were a young boy.** You see, we are talking about basic human needs that have always existed – not something new that is trending now on Twitter.

Do you need to feel nurtured?

If you are missing that feeling of being cared for and looked after, it may be something you have never really experienced. That being the case, you probably don't know how to nurture others. We need to learn from an early age how to do this, and, as a boy, it was probably not one of the skills you were expected to pick up. That being the case, you won't know how to nurture yourself either.

You can begin to do so by paying attention to your feelings and needs. For example, when you get a cut on your hand, you put a bandaid on it, right? In the same way, you need to take care of your emotional wounds by being gentle on yourself and taking the time to heal.

Do you need to express yourself?

It may be extremely difficult for you to open up and express what is going on inside you, yet, you are desperate to talk to someone.

As you know, a problem shared is a problem halved. If your upbringing didn't encourage talking things through or having heart-to-hearts, it's normal to be struggling now to open up.

It won't help that you have been down-talking yourself for years, with that negative inner voice I mentioned in the previous chapter being the only voice you constantly hear.

While changing those negative thought processes can take some time, there are many trained professionals available to help you. That might sound like something only women do and, yes, you are right.

They have usually been brought up to express how they feel, but that doesn't mean you aren't allowed to do the same.

If you have a good friend, why not try opening up to them? You might be surprised to see how desperate they are to express their feelings too but never felt it was the thing to do.

Do you need to feel loved?

It's ok to admit it – you are human after all. From the moment you come into this world, you need to feel secure, nourished and cared for. In other words, you need to feel loved so you can grow into a healthy human being.

Sometimes we don't receive that love when we are young, or not enough of it. This can leave us feeling insecure, vulnerable, and unable to fully connect with others in our adult relationships.

You might have experienced some kind of rejection when you were a kid – maybe from a girl you liked who turned you down. It could be that you were bullied at school, never made the soccer team, or were humiliated by a teacher. All of these negative life experiences go on to shape who you are today.

Painful emotions can stay with you for a very long time, even affecting the way you interact with others. Instead of being open, you might feel closed, protecting yourself at any cost. You still need love, but you don't know how to experience relationships in a healthy way.

Learning to process these past experiences and putting them into perspective is an important part of mastering self-love. This applies to everyone, and not just to men, although you have to begin by getting over the idea that self-love isn't something you are into.

Real men versus good men

Instead of saying, 'Real men don't do that', ask yourself, 'What do good men do?". There is a big difference between the two. The 'real man' is what society has created, and possibly how your parents raised you to be. It's the tough guy: the one who is aggressive, strong, successful, confident, and so on.

A 'good man' is someone with values like integrity and honesty. It's the man who isn't afraid to show emotions and who is nurturing and affectionate. Which one do you really want to be?

All of the 'real man' labels I talked about above put a lot of pressure on men. Not being strong, good at sports, or a born leader can lead to negative feelings about your self-worth if you follow the 'real man' model. On the other hand, when we talk about what being a 'good man' means, things like *dependable, loyal, honest,* and *compassionate* come up. There are qualities a 'real man' isn't supposed to have so when they do come up, you might be worried that they are a sign of your inability to be the man society expects you to be – aggressive, loud, uncaring, and so on.

It is possible, and much more healthy, to be a good man without feeling shame or fear. In his book The Descent of Man[3], Grayson

Perry talks about the masculinity police, who put pressure on boys and men to constantly prove they are a 'real man', which they try to do out of fear of being seen as weak or 'emasculated'.

This is a social norm and it's good to remember that you do not have to fit into that box.

Instead of feeling like you have to be one way or the other, you could shift your perspective a little about what you think masculinity is. There are a lot of great role models out there you can look to: people like David Beckham (a tough soccer player but a loving family man) or Barack Obama (the powerful ex-president of the US who was also intelligent and sensitive). I'll get onto the importance of role models in the next chapter but, for now, I want you to think about who your own role models are and why you look up to them.

If, let's say, your role model is a family member:

- What is it about them that you admire?
- What qualities do they have?
- Why do you want to be like them?
- What qualities do you feel you don't have that they do?
- How can you learn from them?

If you don't have a role model at the moment, choose two or three qualities from the list below you think would make you a better man – a good man:

Loyalty

Honesty

Integrity

Tenderness

Resilience

Calmness

Patience

Courage

Responsibility

Altruism

The above qualities are not only something men should strive for. When talking about 'good men' we are really talking about a good person, so that takes gender out of the equation.

But, unfortunately, men are becoming more and more locked into gender stereotypes. There are definitely differences between men and women, and masculinity is an important aspect of who you are as a man.

The problem many men like you are facing today is that these 'masculine' stereotypes are becoming rigid and harmful. I mentioned earlier in this book about the poor state of men's mental health and higher numbers of suicides than women.

If you are struggling to live up to the external pressures placed on you to be someone you are not, it can seriously affect your emotional well-being.

When you cultivate positive qualities like taking on responsibility and being caring and loyal, you will discover that you feel more whole, grounded, and sure of yourself. There are many ways to be a man, so find the way that suits you and makes you feel proud of yourself.

Instead of believing you have to be thick-skinned, uncaring, and aggressive, embrace positive masculinity. This includes qualities like courage, resilience, and being protective of others – all very masculine strengths you can develop over time.

You can begin by thinking about what changes you can make in the way you think and behave. It's not an overnight process, but if you seriously want to feel better about yourself, you have to start somewhere. Here are some ways you can do so:

1. Love yourself

I am always going to put this at the top of any list because it is the most important thing you can do. When you make a mistake, forgive yourself. When you are tempted to act badly, remember your self-respect. Write down your strengths and weaknesses and accept you are human, not perfect by any means. Celebrate your achievements, follow your passions, take care of your mind and body, and hang out with people who are a positive influence on you.

2. Pursue your ambitions

Want to build your own kit car or get that new promotion? Set yourself goals to achieve this and constantly refine them as you go along. If you want to work less and spend more time with the family, think of how you can achieve this and work toward it. Always keep looking up and ahead instead of down and behind you. This is how dreams come true.

3. Keep your word

When you commit to a project, a plan, or a person, you have to keep your word. Not only will this prove that you do what you say and earn respect, but it will fill you with great satisfaction and increase your self-respect. Don't make promises you know you can't keep as this is no good to anyone. It is ok to say, "No, I can't do what you ask," and this does not make you a failure. It means you are being honest and that's a brave thing to do.

4. Think before you act

It's easy to fly off the handle in a bout of anger and express negative emotions like jealousy and hate. Dissolving these reactions by changing your beliefs about yourself is crucial here. When wild animals feel trapped or scared, they lash out. You don't need to do that and, instead, can work through what is triggering you to react in this way.

Take a second to breathe and focus on why you are feeling this way. Watch the emotion flare up and then let it extinguish itself without any damage done.

5. Own up to your responsibilities

Being responsible isn't about taking something on and then blaming others when things go wrong. It's about being accountable and *not being afraid to say*, "Yep, I didn't do my bit and I have to take the blame for that." When you take on responsibility, make a commitment to yourself to handle it, instead of making excuses about why it didn't work out.

6. Show respect and earn it back

I read somewhere that you can measure the worth of a man by how well he treats people worse off than him. The CEO of a company isn't going to earn the respect of his employees if he walks all over them and why should they? Successful people respect themselves but also show respect for others and can become positive role models.

If you don't feel you are being respected, you need to consider why this is. It could be that you are not earning that respect because you allow people to take advantage of you. Work out what your boundaries are yet still be respectful to others if you wish to command respect in return.

7. Stop judging other people

You never know what someone might be going through or where they are coming from. Instead of being overly critical and putting yourself above them, remove judgment and exercise understanding. Your views may be different from theirs, and that is fine – we can't all agree on everything.

Know where you stand and act based on your principles instead of wasting time down-talking others. Life is too short for that.

8. Learn to be yourself

Explore the qualities you have as a person and be proud of those. Think of ways you can improve and work toward that with a clear vision.

Want to be able to express yourself more? Find an activity that allows you to do that and nurture your creative side. Resist outside pressure to be this way or that – you are unique so be happy and love yourself for that.

And finally, be manly.

Act with determination, strength, confidence, honesty, and integrity.

Be brave enough to take on challenges and strong enough to accept defeat gracefully.

Be fearless in the face of difficulties and know where your limits lie.

Be a good man and make that young boy still inside of you a happy one!

Highlights

- **We all have to grow up and that is often a difficult process for many men.**
- **Parents raise boys differently from how they raise girls, even if they are not aware of it.**
- **Men are put into a box and supposed to portray certain stereotypical masculine qualities.**
- **Boys and men need to feel nurtured, loved, and able to communicate how they feel.**
- **There is a difference between being a 'real man' and being a 'good man'.**
- **Self-love grows when you respect yourself and others, pursue your ambitions, keep your word, take accountability, think before you act, and stop judging others.**
- **Being yourself and creating your own definition of masculinity will make you happier.**

3
BIG BOYS DO CRY

"Cry. Forgive. Learn. Move on. Let your tears water the seeds of your future happiness." – Steve Maraboli

Christian Renaldo is an extremely talented and successful soccer player who has played for some of the biggest teams in Europe. It's not uncommon to see this mighty sportsman moved to tears ... tears of both joy and sorrow.

The Portuguese player literally broke down in tears during a recent interview after seeing a video of his father, who died in 2005. It's touching to watch a grown man crumble before your very eyes, especially a megastar in the world of sport. In fact, many sporting champions have been known to shed a tear or two after winning or losing a big game. And despite those emotional episodes, they still hold nothing but the deepest respect from their fans.

You can watch the Renaldo video on the link below, which has received over 734,000 views so far. Be warned – you may need to get the hankies out.

https://youtu.be/c77HKCYq9XE

The reason I mention Renaldo is that, in many ways, he represents the perfect image of the successful, tough, modern man. He is a role model for millions of youngsters and soccer fans all over the world, but he is also a man who isn't afraid to show his feelings and cry when he gets emotional. He's not the first celebrity to have been filmed crying in public and hopefully, he won't be the last.

Crying is a normal physical reaction and there is absolutely nothing wrong with it but most boys are told not to do it from a certain age onward. It does seem to be more acceptable in a sporting setting though, possibly because this is traditionally seen as a male domain where it's ok to get emotional without breaking those restricting gender stereotypes.

All men cry, although most don't do it in public, and many reserve that kind of behavior for solemn occasions such as when a loved one dies or at a funeral. I want to ask you when was the last time you cried and why? You may need some space to think about that.

In the meantime, we can look at how being told not to cry can affect your ability to express emotions, form close connections with others, and undermine your self-esteem.

Babies cry a lot and they have to. It's a survival instinct that tells the parents or carers when they are hungry, uncomfortable, or in need of soothing. As toddlers grow and develop, they learn to self-soothe but will still cry when in pain, distress, or for attention, amongst other things.

This is all normal childhood behavior and if a child never cried, then there could be something wrong that would need looking into.

At some point though, as boys grow older, they are often told not to cry when they are in pain or feel upset. They might even be told *not to be such a girl*, and to *take it like a man*. The parents are unconsciously or deliberately doing two things here:

- telling their sons to suppress their genuine emotions
- telling them how 'real men' behave

The boy typically grows up thinking that expressing such emotions is a sign of weakness and by the time he reaches his teens, he is an expert at pushing his feelings down.

While the massive hormonal changes he goes through during adolescence can make him behave very erratically, take more risks, and come across as angry, he still doesn't openly show other emotions like pain or sadness.

You might have grown up just like this, with anger being the only 'acceptable' emotion to vent. After all, most teenagers are angry, confused, and frustrated, right? We expect them to throw tantrums and be argumentative so seeing them get angry is all part of that awkward adolescent phase that they are going through.

Because you have learned to hold down your feelings really well, this can make it incredibly difficult for you to form strong emotional bonds with others as you reach adulthood. That makes sense because relationships are built on the sharing of emotions. You might find it easier to open up to a girl or woman than you do with your male friends because they were also probably brought up to believe that doing so is a sign of weakness.

If that's the case, how do you form strong friendships with people who will support you when you need them?

Many men could benefit from mental health treatment to help them deal with these issues of isolation and the inability to bond with others but the truth is that they don't seek that support easily. If and when they do ask for help, men have poor outcomes after treatment compared to women.

This is often because they find it difficult to undo all of the conditioning they experienced about what a 'real man' is or isn't so go into the therapy a bit skeptical from day one. These feelings of loneliness, hostility, and depression that are a result of preconceived gender norms mean that men are stuck between a rock and a hard place. They want to break free but don't know how.

Why crying is good for you

I want to ask you again —when was the last time you cried?

Crying is a natural process that serves several different purposes. We might cry for help, to relieve pain, form and strengthen social bonds, and process emotions. It makes sense that if you never cry, or restrict how much you cry, you could be harming your health in the long run.

We know there are different kinds of tears and they each have an important bodily function. There are:

- Basal tears: fluid produced by your tear ducts to make sure your eyes are kept lubricated
- Reflex tears: these are produced when you get something in your eyes like dust or smoke
- Emotional tears: these flush stress hormones and toxins out of your body

According to The American Academy of Ophthalmology, emotional tears contain hormones that stimulate the release of cortisol, which is the stress hormone in your body.

Crying is a self-soothing behavior that activates the parasympathetic nervous system. This enables you to relax after a time of stress, much like taking the top off a valve to release all of that built-up pressure.

When you suppress emotions, you're not giving yourself the chance to feel and process them, no matter whether they are negative or positive. Apart from that, emotional crying releases oxytocin and endorphins, the hormones responsible for soothing pain and helping you to feel better.

What happens when you keep everything bottled up?

If you feel like you can't show how you feel and tend to repress your emotions, this can eventually affect your physical well-being. Repressive coping, as it is technically called, can lead to health conditions such as:

- cancer

- cardiovascular diseases, including hypertension (high blood pressure)
- lower immune system function

Studies carried out in 2013[1] and 2018[2] showed a link between repressing emotions and a range of physiological illnesses, like depression and stress. When the participants of the study who said they didn't cry anymore were asked to fill in a questionnaire, 46.1% of them reported feeling less:

- social connection
- social support
- empathy

I hope this helps you to understand that not only do you have permission to cry, but you should do it as often as you feel the need. If you want to practice self-love, you need to look after your physical and mental welfare and crying is a very good way to do that.

No matter what social conditioning you have undergone or how you were brought up, the facts speak for themselves – crying is good for you. The only time it would be worrying is if you find yourself crying uncontrollably and feel weepy all the time for no apparent reason. This could suggest depression and it would do you the world of good to talk to a therapist if that is the case.

Toxic masculinity

I have to talk to you about the phenomenon of toxic masculinity that has grown over the past few years because it may be affecting you. It's an attitude promoted mainly across social media platforms but also in movies, music, and books by men who feel disillusioned with their lives.

You might not have heard the term 'toxic masculinity' before, but I am sure you will recognize it when I describe it. It's the narrow and repressive description of manhood, defined by violence, sex, status, success, and aggression. It's this idea that to be a man, you need to be strong. Emotions are a weakness and your worth is measured by how violent you are. Sex and brutality are part of the agenda, and it's ok to blame women for your problems and mistreat them.

Many outspoken influencers are taking advantage of this disillusionment among young men and inciting misogyny and violence. This is a serious downturn that has given rise to dangerous subcultures like INCEL, which stands for 'involuntary celibate'.

The INCEL culture puts resentment, misogyny, self-pity, and self-loathing at the top of its agenda. There is also a sense of entitlement to sex and the endorsement of violence against women and sexually active people.

While these ideas might not resonate with you in any way, you could still feel that your discontentment has something to do with women and your inability to have a successful relationship with them.

Now is a good time to think about how you see women and if those perceptions are feeding the discontentment you feel about yourself.

You might be struggling with unemployment, poor housing, lack of money, and poverty. Finding friends or a partner may seem hard, and you could spend a lot of time alone feeling frustrated and unhappy.

Your peers might be in the same position as you and your life doesn't seem to be moving in the direction you want it to.

Bad experiences with women may have left you with a bunch of negative emotions such as rejection and humiliation. It's even possible that you feel lost and have very low self-esteem.

With the online world replacing authentic social interactions, there is a danger that you can absorb damaging opinions without realizing it, especially if you tune into a lot of the toxic masculinity narratives out there.

Women have been oppressed for far too long and are now more motivated than ever to succeed. This shift has caused a lot of men to feel threatened, or even obsolete, which is not a healthy development for anyone.

Breaking the negative cycle

If you are a young man and you're struggling, I want to tell you that you are not alone. But you can help yourself out of this phase of your life and move on to better things. I want to help you to rethink your approach to life and create a new mindset that will fill you with a greater amount of self-worth and self-esteem. Here are some powerful ways to do that:

- **Learn self-awareness**

Self-awareness is a crucial step to understanding your emotions and working through your problems. It's a kind of unlearning process in a way. Instead of accepting the way you are, take time to think about things differently. Are the emotions and thoughts you experience really coming from your authentic self, or are they layers of conditioning piled on top of you over the years?

Allow yourself to experience your feelings instead of blocking them out. The next time you feel hurt, inspect that feeling like you would if you caught a bug in your hand. What does it look like?

Where did it come from? What triggered it? Try to think of the last time you felt the same way – are there any similarities between then and now? And finally, allow yourself to experience that emotion like you were surfing a wave.

Notice how long it takes before it subsides and consider how you feel when it has lost its energy. Cry if you feel like it and wash away any tension or stress that has been building up. When you are in tune with your emotions, you are in a much better position to process and understand them.

Follow your instincts. This means stopping to listen whenever your gut feeling tells you something is not right about your behavior. When you do things that go against your better nature, your inner self is telling you this is not right so stay tuned to that voice. It will never let you down.

Identify what activities genuinely make you happy. If you love swimming, for example, what exactly is it that you love so much? Is it the sense of freedom, the sensation of the water on your skin, or the challenge of stretching your physical capabilities? Make a list of 5 things you love to do such as my example below:

hanging out with your buddies

going kayaking

playing basketball

dancing

Bowling

Try to do at least one of these things each week and invite your friends to join you. Do more of what you love and enjoy life to the fullest.

Expand your horizons. Get to know the world around you better instead of living in your bedroom. There is a lot to explore, from different cultures to new landscapes. You might not be able to afford to travel but you can walk around your neighborhood and see it from a different perspective.

Try out new food you've never tasted before, go see a movie you would never normally watch, join a book club, or start learning how to play a new instrument. Get out and discover life instead of sitting in your room and complaining.

Act with love. I have no doubt that you love your family and friends, but you might not show them that often. Remember that self-love means being brave enough to express how you feel and there's no better place to start than with loved ones.

Hug your dad more often (he might be surprised but will enjoy it), make time for a friend who is going through a bad patch, or do more housework instead of leaving it all to your partner. The love you receive is always equal to the love you give so go for it and show how much you care with actions, not words.

Stop playing video games. This might be an unpopular suggestion, but it's worth considering anyway. Video games are great and there's no doubt about that. They are fun, exciting, challenging, and a wonderful escape from reality. I'm a big fan of online games but I also know that spending too much time playing has some negative side effects.

The main one is that you can become too disengaged from real-world pursuits, which isn't healthy. As a social animal, you need to be interacting in real contexts and not through a screen. At least try to limit the time you play to an hour a day and do something else with friends and family.

Get physical. Sitting at a desk all day in front of a PC or TV are not good outlets for your need for physical stimulation. You need intensive physical activity to activate healthy levels of testosterone, which has several positive effects. Go for a half-hour run each day, follow a workout routine that suits you, or join a local sports team. Once you get going, you can reap the benefits of:

Fat loss

Muscle gain

Healthier bone density

Normalized blood pressure

Less likelihood of obesity and heart attacks

Increased energy

More enjoyment of life

Feeling more positive

Healthy sex drive

Increased motivation

Improved focus

Better memory

Put regular exercise in your life and see what a difference it makes in how you feel after just one week. You will be amazed!

Learn a new skill. Whenever you learn something new, it will give you a great sense of achievement and boost your self-esteem. It could be anything from learning coding to Japanese – whatever takes your fancy.

You could have a lot of untapped talent just waiting to be discovered so set some time aside each week to learn a new craft and give yourself a pat on the back!

Finally, I want you to imagine you are talking to your younger self. Think of how you would treat him when you see him in pain, hurt, and upset. It's a nice exercise to create that dialogue in your mind and allows your younger self to benefit from your care and compassion.

Tell him you understand his fears, uncertainties, and disappointment and that it's ok to cry.

Acknowledge the challenges he is facing and that it's ok to be vulnerable.

Tell him it's ok to ask for help.

Hug him and let him know you are there for him.

When you embrace that young boy you once were, you are nourishing yourself and that's a wonderful way to develop self-love.

Highlights

- **Many male celebrities and sportsmen have been caught crying on camera, and are still respected by their fans.**
- **Crying is a natural response to pain, sorrow, and stress that can do you the world of good.**
- **Repressing your emotions can have long-term health effects on your mind and body.**
- **Toxic masculinity won't make you feel better about yourself. It will only fuel negativity and hate.**
- **You can break the negative thought cycle by adopting a new mindset.**
- **Self-awareness is key to understanding why you react the way you do.**
- **Paying attention to your feelings is healthier than blocking them out.**

- **When you follow your gut instinct, it will take you in the right direction.**
- **Expand your horizons, learn a new skill, and look after your body if you want to feel better about yourself.**
- **Share love through simple actions and receive more love in return.**
- **Spend less time playing video games and more time pursuing the things you love with real people.**
- **Embrace your inner child and show him how much you love him.**

4
MEN WHO HURT OTHERS ARE OFTEN HURT THEMSELVES

"Trauma is the invisible force that shapes our lives. It shapes the way we live, the way we love, and the way we make sense of the world. It is the root of our deepest wounds." –Gabor Maté

Everybody can give and receive love, although many people find that hard to do. They may have been hurt in the past and have become distrustful of others ever since then. The child who is neglected or abused by his parents/carers could still be carrying around a lot of emotional pain.

The emotional wounds often go untreated for a very long time and never heal. They translate into problems such as low self-esteem, guilt, social anxiety, depression, and the inability to form meaningful relationships.

Some people deal with those painful wounds by adopting a self-defense mechanism where they will hurt others before being hurt again themselves.

This could be in the form of bullying, gaslighting, manipulation, coercion, or any other kind of emotional and physical abuse. Not everyone reacts in this way of course, although the statistics show that someone who has suffered trauma in early life is more likely to display this kind of behavior.

Masculinity and violence

According to the Office for National Statistics UK[1], violence against women by men is on the rise, with domestic abuse, sexual assault, and murder becoming more frequent. The majority (60%) of female murder victims knew their killer personally, with a third of the suspects being current or former partners.

These are frightening figures, but it doesn't mean that all men are violent by nature. Many men also fall victim to violent crimes, domestic violence, coercion, and sexual abuse. In the US, male victimization is a big public health problem, with the results of the National Intimate Partner and Sexual Violence Survey (NISVS)[2] showing nearly a quarter of men reported some form of contact sexual violence in their lifetime.

Incidents of sexual and physical violence seriously impact the victims for a long time afterward, who can suffer from fear and post-traumatic stress disorder as a result.

Violence has nothing to do with the Y chromosome or being macho. Just because you are a man, this doesn't make you prone to violence. Experts agree that what makes men more likely to commit such crimes are things like individual characteristics, environmental factors, upbringing, exposure to neglect, and maltreatment in their early years.

Different stressors in life can produce anger and frustration, which may lead to violence. Male victims are more likely to react violently to such strains or triggers, while women victims tend to internalize their responses. As a man, if you have grown up in a culture where expressing emotions is considered to be unmasculine and there is pressure to conform to certain expectations of dominance and aggression, this might lead you to behave violently[3].

Many men behave aggressively when they experience stress that comes from a self-perceived failure to live up to masculine expectations. Violence within an intimate partnership shows the feelings of distress males experience when they feel their idealized masculine identity is being threatened[4].

Often though, the incidents of violence that take place within homes and between couples are much more subtle and often go undetected for a very long time.

Most of us feel bad when we hurt others because we are social beings by nature and would never intentionally hurt someone's feelings, never mind being physically abusive with them. You hear the words 'narcissist' and 'sociopath' being thrown around a lot, but these labels don't apply to everyone.

Being mean to your girlfriend doesn't necessarily make you a sociopath, but it could suggest you have some issues you need to work through.

If you do behave in a hurtful way to others, you are probably hurting inside. You might not be aware of that fully, or make excuses for your behavior. Remember that no one is responsible for your behavior apart from you. Apportioning blame to justify your damaging words and actions is not fair and also very cowardly.

How are you feeling?

The way you feel inside is the key to understanding why you behave the way you do. Anger is one of those negative feelings that can be very destructive, especially when it becomes your normal way of being.

Imagine that it's a normal day. You get up, get ready for work, spill your coffee on your shirt, miss the train or get stuck in traffic. When you do get to work, your boss pulls you up about some project you didn't complete on time, and you have to stay past working hours at the end of the day to finish it.

These are all normal events in life – they might suck but they aren't enough to make you lose your cool, right?

You might be a bit peeved, as anyone would be, but do things like this make you feel angry? If so, do you think you might be overreacting and that anger is coming from somewhere else?

What if you go into the red zone whenever another driver cuts in front of you on the freeway, or you get involved in a fight with your girlfriend because she wants to go out with her friends?

When you feel destructive emotions like anger and rage building up inside you, they can become so huge that they strangle more healing emotions like compassion, empathy, and love. Eventually, you will create a monster that you can't control.

When your stomach is churning, you feel on edge, and want to break something, these are all signs that you are not dealing well with anger and hurt in your life.

Fear is another powerful emotion that can stop you from developing healthy relationships with others. It is self-destructive, holding you back from true happiness, and is the cause of a lot of anxiety. You might find it difficult to sleep, concentrate, interact with others, or set goals and will even avoid any situations you think will make you feel vulnerable.

All of these negative emotions can make you say and do things you wouldn't normally do. How many times have you lashed out in anger, spoken harshly to a loved one, lost your temper, or even physically abused someone?

There are times when we all get frustrated and angry, but knowing how to deal with those emotions is important, otherwise, they can get us into a lot of trouble.

Taking back control

When I suggest taking control of your feelings, I don't mean suppressing them. What you need to do is acknowledge them and try to see where they are coming from. Once you do that, you can remove their power over you and take back control of your life. At the moment, you might be acting more like a runaway train on a collision course and that is not what you want.

Here's a simple test. Ask yourself these four questions:

1. What am I feeling right now?

2. Why am I feeling it?
3. What would make me feel better in this situation?
4. What is a healthy way to express how I'm feeling?

Every time you feel like you are overreacting or being triggered by something that has happened, stop and ask yourself the four questions above. As you do so, consider the following points:

- Identify the feeling and give it a name: is it anger, fear, rage, or jealousy?
- What triggered it – something someone said or did? Something you said or did?
- Can you ease this negative feeling by walking away, taking a few breaths, or going for a run?
- Can you express how you are feeling in a calm, unthreatening way?

This is a kind of self-regulation that will stop you from behaving in a way you might regret later. It's a strategy you can use any time you feel that you are going to lose control. Once you get used to doing it, you will be able to work through negative emotions more successfully without causing damage to yourself or others.

Managing your anger

Anger is a toxic emotion that can be triggered very easily if left to its own devices. We now know that people who feel constantly angry have a lot of underlying issues they need to sort out. Past trauma is one of them, and I'll be looking at that further on in this chapter. For the moment, ask yourself, are you angry because:

- People don't understand you?
- You feel underappreciated and disrespected?
- Your boss, friends, or family members are taking advantage of you?
- Someone you care about has deceived you or lied to you?
- Anything else?

Whatever the reasons for your feelings of anger, you need to find out what is behind it. Use this guideline to help you:

Feeling misunderstood can make you feel like you don't count and are worthless. When did you last feel the same way? What happened then and how hurt were you when you experienced it?

Feeling underappreciated can be linked to low levels of self-esteem. When did you last feel the same way? What happened then and how hurt were you when you experienced it?

Feeling you are being taken advantage of could be linked to an abusive relationship in the past, where your feelings were not considered. When did you last feel the same way? What happened then and how hurt were you when you experienced it?

Feeling betrayed or lied to could be linked to a time in the past when someone you trusted let you down badly. When did you last feel the same way? What happened then and how hurt were you when you experienced it?

Ignoring the reasons why you react the way you do is only going to give more power to those destructive emotions. Instead of dealing with them, you are burying them deeper and deeper into your psyche until you want to explode.

You can detect the signs that you are going to lose it before things get out of control and they usually go something like this:

- You begin shouting and getting verbally abusive
- You make sarcastic, nasty comments
- You get a stomachache, headache, or feel tension in your neck and shoulders.
- You begin to have aggressive thoughts
- You have the urge to hurt someone
- You experience a choking sensation
- You clench your jaw and fists

Notice how your body reacts to anger – it's as if you are getting into attack mode. As the anger spirals to the fore, your adrenaline pumps at a high rate and you are ready to strike the enemy before they strike you.

This is not the way to handle life and I am sure you know that. But the fact that you are acting this way should be a clear indication that you need to get to the bottom of your issues.

Behaving badly

When you feel worthless, it's easy to put others down so you feel better about yourself. It might give you a feeling of control and power at the expense of a partner or loved one.

The problem with this kind of attitude is that it can lead to damaging and criminal behavior. You will have heard of coercive control and might even be a victim of it yourself (coercive control can happen to both men and women).

Coercion can take many forms and is reinforced by social beliefs that give men the right to dominate their partner (usually a man exerting control over a woman). It can include things like:

- One-sided power games
- Manipulation
- Mind games
- Overprotection and 'caring'
- Isolation
- Degradation
- Humiliation
- Denial
- Blaming
- Economic abuse
- Sexual abuse
- The list goes on...

You can be coercive without actually being physically violent to the victim although it is just as painful. Gaslighting is another kind of control that makes the victim think they are losing their mind. The perpetrator creates doubt in the victim's mind about what happened or what was said to exert power over them.

Like any kind of control, gaslighting makes the perpetrator feel better about their own inadequacies and insecurities. They have also very likely been the victim of the same kind of abuse at the hands of their parents or carers and it's a learned behavior pattern.

If you feel that you are in a coercive relationship, either as a perpetrator or victim, you need to seek help. This is a serious situation that could escalate to extreme violence and tragic consequences and it is not something you should ignore.

As you know, fear doesn't earn respect or love. Negative emotions only breed contempt and feelings of shame and guilt. Understanding your emotions can help you to see what you need to pay attention to. An absence of self-esteem and self-respect doesn't develop overnight and it also takes time to deal with these issues. Be patient as you begin to do the self-work you need to overcome your negative reactions to the ones you love.

Working through trauma

We all know that childhood experiences shape our view of the world as we reach adulthood. Even if you have a very happy, safe upbringing, you might have experienced something bad in the past that had a big impact on you.

Your teacher might have scolded you in the front of the class or you could have been bullied by the other kids. Maybe your coach took you off the soccer team because you weren't good enough or you failed to get into university.

Perhaps you experienced domestic violence between your parents or lost someone close to you. You might even have been a victim of crime or caught up in social unrest, even war. All of these examples can be very traumatic for anyone and the younger you are, the more likely they are to affect you.

The problem is that if you never make peace with them or resolve them, those feelings of loss, pain and anxiety will stay with you. Dr.

Gabor Maté, a leading health expert, has done a lot of work on the effects of trauma on men and women.

His research shows a clear link between childhood trauma and addiction, stress, and physical illness. I've already mentioned how stress can affect your health and now I want you to think about how past traumas might be blocking your ability to be happy today.

When you were hurt in some way, you probably started to build a kind of mental armor to protect yourself from further harm. Instead of seeking help or therapy to overcome what you went through, you locked it away in a box and threw away the key. It is just too hurtful to face, right?

The harder you get, the more difficult it will be for you to give and receive love, even though that is what you crave. Acting as if you are tough and never being vulnerable can hurt people around you, who think you are uncaring and insensitive. Most importantly of all, you are hurting yourself because you aren't living to the full and enjoying every dimension of life. Feelings like resentment, bitterness, and sadness can fester, which are toxic to your emotional well-being.

If you can open that box (you might need a sledgehammer) and get rid of whatever has been weighing you down for so long, you can level up in your life.

You could be protecting yourself from pain through resignation. This is when you say things like, "I can't be bothered, nothing is going to change, I am who I am...' If you catch yourself saying any of these, you could be distancing yourself from people and not showing them you care about them.

This leads to social isolation at the end of the day, and you might be experiencing that right now.

You have so much power to turn things around but you need to change the narrative. Instead of saying, 'It is what it is,' **say,**

My past doesn't define my present.

I will show that I care.

I can change for the better.

You could be defending yourself from pain through defiance. You might say things like "I don't need anyone else, I can do it alone, no one is going to tell me what to do." You probably don't want to be put in the position of feeling vulnerable or helpless and can become withdrawn or give people the silent treatment.

Even though you feel threatened when you think anything is robbing you of your self-sufficiency, you show contempt when you see someone close to you being vulnerable.

You have to put down your weapons and admit you feel vulnerable sometimes, which is OK. Everyone needs someone and you can only experience a close bond with another person when you are emotionally open. **Say:**

I do need someone in my life.

I can't do everything alone.

I will ask for help.

You could be defending yourself from pain through compromise. You could say things like, "I will only risk it if you risk it too." This might sound reasonable but what you are actually doing is demanding that someone else has to prove themselves first. No matter how often they do that, it will never be enough for you and that other person will feel they can never do enough.

If you want to have a healthy relationship, you have to give 100% and hope the other person will too. You probably use this kind of thinking about yourself too, doing things half-heartedly because you don't think you will succeed. This will make you feel discontent and unsatisfied with life in general.

Instead of compromise, be fully present in anything you do without expectations or fear of failure. **Say:**

I will do whatever it takes.

Every day I am getting better and better.

I will give it my best shot.

You might be defending yourself through cowardice. This is when you say things like, "I'll do whatever it takes to protect myself from being exposed." This is a tactic you use to avoid experiencing the feeling of being vulnerable to pain.

It's your way of defending yourself because you are still carrying around pain from something that happened to you in the past. As you block the process of healing your emotional wounds, you are also sabotaging your chances of happiness.

Instead of protecting yourself, gently examine where that pain is coming from. Understand that it happened TO you and it is NOT who you are. **Say:**

I am brave enough to face my pain.

I can move on from the past and enjoy the present.

My future is in my hands.

When you have reached a point in your life where you cannot see the light at the end of the tunnel, take strength from the power you have within you. If you are willing to change, you will find the courage to do so. It can be scary opening up and risk being hurt again but the alternative is not going to help you.

The process of change comes through recognizing what has been holding you back and allowing yourself to get closer to your authentic self. You will discover a lot of love buried under all the baggage and realize just how wonderful it is to let it flow.

Highlights

- **Violence is not a trait of masculinity. It's a social construct adopted by some men.**
- **Ask yourself how you feel and examine those negative emotions to find out where they come from.**
- **Take control of your life instead of letting it control you.**

- **Identify when you are feeling angry and learn how to diffuse it.**
- **Change your behavior when it is hurting others and seek help if you find yourself a victim of abuse.**
- **Work through trauma by lowering your defenses and opening up.**

/ 5 /

SAY GOODBYE TO LOW SELF-ESTEEM FOR GOOD

"If you put a small value upon yourself, rest assured that the world will not raise your price." – Author Unknown

You probably know one or two guys who just seem to ooze self-confidence from every pore. They are the ones who always look great and are successful, popular, funny, smart, and cool to be around.

And then you go and look in the mirror and convince yourself you aren't that handsome, don't consider yourself to be successful, wouldn't say you were that popular, and don't believe that you are much fun to hang out with.

Well, that's the perception you have of yourself, right? We are what we tell ourselves we are so if you feel unattractive or boring, it's difficult to convince you otherwise.

The thing is, that negative preconception you have about yourself is very damaging, even if you might not be aware of it. In your head, you have formed a picture of who you are that could be totally false. But because you have bought into it and think it is the 'real you', you are letting it control your life.

More often than not, this perception of yourself has developed over time because of your low self-esteem and that is something I want to talk about with you in this chapter. You have probably never heard any of your male friends saying, 'I have low self-esteem'... it's not something men are supposed to admit to, is it?

But many thousands of men ARE suffering from low self-esteem, and that has a massive impact on the way they behave and how they handle their lives.

What is self-esteem?

Self-esteem is basically the opinion you have of yourself. If you like yourself and value your achievements, then we can say that you have a healthy level of self-esteem. If, on the other hand, you don't like yourself, or feel dissatisfied and unhappy about who you are most of the time, then you probably have low levels of self-esteem.

Why is self-esteem important?

Not liking yourself, for whatever reason, means you are never going to feel happy. Instead of enjoying life, you will be constantly putting yourself down and limiting your potential to thrive. This has a damaging effect on your relationships, your job or career, as well as your own mental and physical health.

We might all go through rough patches in our lives when we feel unworthy, although these thoughts usually disappear once we pick ourselves up again.

But if you have suffered from low-self esteem for a long time, it can be much harder to change your mindset and start to like yourself again. You might be wondering if you are really suffering from low self-esteem, so take a look at the points below and see if you can relate to any of them.

Characteristics of low self-esteem

You are extremely critical of yourself (*I'm useless*)

You downplay or ignore your positive qualities (*I'm not that good at sport*)

You judge yourself to be inferior to your peers (*I'm not as successful as Joe*)

You use negative words to describe yourself, such as dumbass, idiot, flabby, undesirable (*I'm such a deadbeat*)

Your self-talk is always negative, critical and self blaming (*I keep making stupid mistakes*)

You assume that your achievements are down to luck and don't take the credit for them (*I just got lucky, that's all*)

You automatically blame yourself when things go wrong (*I messed up again*)

You don't believe someone when they compliment you (*They are just saying that and don't really mean it*)

When your self-esteem is at a low, it doesn't matter what other people say: your idea of yourself is fixed in concrete and nobody can dig you out if it.

I can tell you how funny, smart, attractive, and worthy you are until the cows come home but if you don't believe it yourself, my words will fall on deaf ears. That is why only you can increase your positive feelings about who you are and what you are capable of, although I can give you a helping hand if you are ready.

How is low self-esteem affecting your life?

You might have never thought about self-esteem and how it is affecting your life. If you haven't made that connection between your behavior and its consequences, now is a good time to reconnect the dots and consider how your low self-esteem is affecting everything you do.

Negative feelings – Do you have any negative emotions about yourself? When you constantly self-criticize and put yourself down, this is going to create persistent feelings of sadness, depression, anxiety, anger, shame or guilt.

Relationship problems – Do you feel like a victim or perpetrator in your relationships? Low self-esteem is a recipe for disaster because it makes you put up with unreasonable behavior and can even lead you to take your anger and frustration out on your partner.

Fear of trying – Do you feel trapped by your own self-doubt? If you don't believe in your abilities, you are less likely to try out new things, step outside of your comfort zone, or take on challenges.

Perfectionism – Do you push yourself to the limit in an attempt to achieve perfection? If you think you have to be perfect all the time or over-achieve, this could be an unconscious response to deeper feelings of being inferior or 'not good enough'.

Fear of judgment – Do you avoid any situations where you might be criticized or judged? If you purposefully shy away from any activity that involves other people because you are afraid you will be negatively judged, you are allowing your low-self esteem to sabotage your life.

Low resilience – Do you find it difficult to cope with challenging life events? If you believe that you are hopeless, you will not find it easy to handle simple everyday problems and will give up control to someone else.

Lack of self-care – Do you drink too much, use drugs, smoke, or indulge in any other unhealthy habits? If your self-esteem is at rock bottom, you won't take care of yourself and will end up doing more damage to your physical and emotional health in the long run.

What is normal?

After reading the above effects of low self-esteem, how many seem normal to you and how many seem abnormal? For example, do you think it is acceptable that you avoid playing sports because you don't want to be called a bad player?

Is it OK to place all the responsibilities on your partner or family instead of helping just because you believe you aren't capable of handling them?

If any of the above seem like 'normal' behavior to you, it might be a sign that you are really suffering from low self-esteem and it's important to identify that if it is the case.

Once you understand that a lot of your behavior is linked to how you see yourself, you will realize that your 'present normal' is not necessarily how you should be living – you can create a 'new normal' that reflects the real you. Here are some things to think about in relation to how you feel:

- Are you often told that you are over-sensitive to criticism?
- Do you avoid social gatherings and prefer to self-isolate?
- Do you continually have negative thoughts about yourself or your abilities?
- Do you find it difficult to assert yourself?
- Do you have trouble making eye contact or maintaining a confident posture?

If you answered yes to some or all of the above, my guess is that you really don't like yourself too much, if at all. For whatever reason (and I'll come to those in a little while), you have let yourself slide into a narrative of self-doubt and self-criticism.

It is a lot easier to reject people, hide away, and feel bad than it is to start believing in yourself. That takes courage, guts, and willpower – all things you have forgotten how to do but hope is not lost. You can overcome all of this negativity and restore your self-esteem once you make the decision to do so.

How are you doing?

To help you get started, I want you to choose one answer from the statements below that reflects how you feel about yourself at this moment. Each statement gives you the choice of saying you **strongly agree** with it, **agree, disagree,** or **strongly disagree.** Let's take a look and see how you go:

I feel like I have as much worth as others.

Strongly agree

Agree

Disagree

Strongly disagree

On the whole, I am satisfied with myself.

Strongly agree

Agree

Disagree

Strongly disagree

I never feel useless.

Strongly agree

Agree

Disagree

Strongly disagree

I treat myself kindly when things don't go right.

Strongly agree

Agree

Disagree

Strongly disagree

I have several good qualities.

Strongly agree

Agree

Disagree

Strongly disagree

If you chose 'Strongly disagree' to a lot of these questions, you are probably struggling with self-esteem. Now that you know that, you can start to think about where all of this is coming from.

Getting to the root of the problem is always the best way to overcome it, although you will need to spend some time digging until you get there.

What is causing your low self-esteem?

You might have always had low self-esteem ever since growing up, or just recently started to experience it due to certain events in your life. Either way, knowing what triggered it is the best way to deal with it.

The way you feel about yourself is often an idea imposed on you by others that you have come to believe over the years. Maybe your parents or carers made you feel unworthy or unloved. Other times, a rejection from a partner or a failure in your professional life can make you feel worthless.

We all internalize things differently and it is easy to beat ourselves up when things go wrong. If we do this often enough, it can become a bad habit that makes us judge ourselves way too harshly.

Here are some of the common causes of low self-esteem. Can you relate to any of them?

- An unhappy childhood where your parents (or other adults such as teachers) were extremely critical
- Difficulty with your academic performance in school which affected your confidence
- A stressful life event such as relationship breakdown or financial problems
- Being in an abusive relationship with a partner, parent or carer
- Ongoing medical problems such as serious illness or physical disability
- Mental illness like depression or social anxiety disorder

The above are all things that HAPPENED to you. You did not cause them and they do not define who you really are. Let's look at them differently:

Whatever you experienced in childhood, the responsibility lies on the adults – they were the ones who treated you badly. You did not deserve that.

The problems you faced with your school work were not a reflection of your capabilities. They represent an educational system that probably failed you. You need to remember that.

Breakdowns in relationships and financial problems are a part of life. They happen to everyone and even the most successful people can lose out in love or have money worries. It's how you deal with them that counts.

Many people find themselves in abusive relationships, which can erode the confidence of even the most self-assured individuals over time. If you are involved in this kind of relationship, you need to remove yourself from it as soon as possible and seek professional help if you can.

Long-term medical problems and mental health issues can be totally devastating to your emotional wellbeing over time. Here, some self-compassion can help you to find your balance, and you should also seek as much support as possible to help you cope.

Making your low self-esteem worse

Being told you are useless, unworthy, or unattractive will grow into a belief you carry around with you, even if it is not true. If you do have low-self-esteem, this colors the way you look at the world and you might be making yourself feel even worse without realizing it. Some of the bad habits you might have adopted could include:

Comparing yourself to other guys. As a man, you are probably very critical of yourself in comparison to other more 'successful' men. These feelings of inadequacy are self-destructive because instead of telling yourself you are worthy, you believe you aren't as good as someone else.

Dating pressure. There is still a lot of pressure on men to be successful at dating and any bad experiences can leave you feeling insecure about your value as a man. Having to be competitive in the dating pool and trying to live up to cultural expectations of what a 'man' does could leave you feeling stressed and full of anxiety.

Gender stereotyping. Masculine stereotypes can seriously prevent you from being yourself, and this is very damaging for your sense of identity. Whatever your sexual orientation or how you define your gender, if you aren't allowed to express that freely, your self-esteem is going to suffer.

You need to feel comfortable in your own skin and have role models who you can relate to instead of stereotypes that don't represent you.

Mental health issues. As I mentioned earlier, most men find it very hard to seek help when they are suffering from mental health issues. It just isn't 'manly' to admit you are suffering from stress, anxiety, or depression, right? But mental health is just as important as physical health and you need to look after both.

Body image issues. This is a massive problem for many men, who are bombarded with the 'perfect body type' in our appearance-obsessed culture. You might believe you need to have a certain look, body, and lifestyle, otherwise you have less worth as an individual. Of course, these false standards are totally superficial. Looks don't really count for that much: it's what's inside that is important – believe me.

Fear of failure. In a world geared toward success in relationships, careers, and money, failure in any of those can feel like a punch in the gut. Being a 'loser' isn't an option, so when things don't work out, your self-esteem can hit rock bottom. There is always the chance that things don't go as you had planned in life and that doesn't make you a failure.

Lack of validation from others. Your self-worth may be linked to external validation from others about your abilities and achievements. You want to get that pat on the back and hear the words, 'Well done', so when that doesn't happen, you could feel worthless. Self-validation is the key to knowing your worth and hearing it from others is an extra bonus!

Suffering in silence. If you have low self-esteem, you will probably feel sorry for yourself and keep apologizing for your bad behavior but can't share what is going on inside you. No doubt, you are extremely hard on yourself and think you don't deserve to be happy or successful. This is such a sad way to live and means you are missing out on so many joys in life.

Shifting blame. You might even blame everyone else for your predicament and take your frustration out on your partner, friends, family, or even perfect strangers.

By shifting the responsibility to someone else, you are saying, 'I'm not accountable for my actions and feelings.' This is not the mark of a good man – it's the habit of someone who is sticking his head in the sand. Things won't get better until you learn to 'man up' and take back control of your life.

Having a victim mentality. If you feel like a victim, you are giving up your power to live the way you want. You may have gone through something extremely hurtful or traumatic in the past, which makes you still feel vulnerable.

If that's the case, try to put into perspective what you experienced and remember that you don't need to be a victim anymore.

I know it isn't easy to move from a negative mindset to feeling good about yourself. It can take time to get to the root cause and unlearn all the conditioning you have picked up over the years. I want to stress that how you identify yourself today is a remnant of past events and does not reflect the person you really are.

When you get rid of those old labels, you will discover someone who is worthy, able, and capable of so many things. If you stopped trying to achieve anything or pursue your dreams because you think you don't deserve success or happiness, I'm here to tell you to press the restart button. Everyone deserves to lead a fulfilling life no matter what went on in their past – including you.

If you really want to be the kind of man that is admired and looked up to, start by wiping the slate clean and seeing yourself differently.

Each new day is a fresh opportunity to look at yourself in the mirror and say, 'I am just as good as the next man and deserve to be happy.' Once you have learned that morning mantra, let's see how else you can get back that empowering self-esteem.

My top 10 confidence tips

Believe you can make the right decisions. When you lack confidence, it's hard to make decisions because you fear they aren't the right ones. It's easier to sit on the fence and leave the decision-making to someone else but this means you lose your power over what happens in your life. Even making mistakes in the past doesn't mean you will always make mistakes in the future. Think instead of all the small achievements and wins you have made up to today – they prove that you have the intelligence and ability to make sound decisions.

Stop talking down to yourself. Instead of repeating the criticisms others have made about you, remind yourself of your strengths. I am sure you can do quite a few things really well, have some awesome qualities, and can even boast a unique skill set. I want you to name 3 positive things about yourself here and now... anything at all. Take on the challenge and note 3 things that you can be proud of.

Embrace your mistakes. It takes more guts to say, 'I messed up' than it does to deny it. We all feel bad when we slip up but the wisdom lies in learning from that and moving on. Mistakes help us to grow and mature, giving us the experience we need to do better next time. Even if you feel embarrassed, acknowledging where you went wrong is the key to improvement.

Owning your mistakes will make you stronger and better equipped to do the right thing in the future. See mistakes as life's lessons and not eternal punishment!

Be grateful. You might think you have nothing to be grateful for, but think again. Good things could be all around you and you never notice them because you focus too much on the negatives. Do you have your health, a job, a partner, or a good friend? You can be grateful for all of these.

Even the ability to breathe, walk, see the sunrise, smell the coffee – every single thing in life is a gift. Ask yourself what you are grateful for and you will instantly feel better about yourself.

Take a look in the mirror. When was the last time you looked in the mirror and liked what you saw? A lot of the time, we see a distorted view of ourselves when we gaze into our reflection. Our eyes immediately go to all of those imperfections – a crooked nose, spotty complexion, big chin... and so on.

But look again, this time saying something positive about yourself like, 'I have a great head of hair, my eyes are a cool color, I look great for my age....' Find at least one positive thing to say about yourself and shake off all the negativity you have been carrying around with you.

Accept change. You aren't the same man you were yesterday and will have changed again by tomorrow. Life is like that: a constant series of changes where nothing is permanent. That means you can be better, stronger, more balanced, and happier if you set yourself goals to work toward.

Instead of being stuck in the same old rut you are in, think about what you can do to create positive change in your life, starting today. Can you eat healthier and work out more? Can you change your inner dialogue from a negative one to a positive one? Can you tend to your deep emotional needs and find time for self-care?

Believe in your self-worth. A confident man knows that his happiness is important and that he's worthy of it. If you want to have more success, money, or romance in your life, you must believe you deserve it.

This will give you the motivation to pursue those dreams with greater momentum and discover it is possible to achieve them. Your self-worth doesn't lie in your race, ethnicity, sexual orientation, or gender – we are all worthy of happiness, no matter what!

Look after yourself. It is crucial that you practice self-care and if you don't do it, no one else will do it for you. You might find it difficult to put the time and energy into improving your appearance but it will definitely boost your self-confidence.

There's nothing girly about having a skincare routine, being well-groomed, or smelling clean. And if you look good on the outside, you will feel good on the inside too!

Embrace your imperfections. You know that it's the imperfections that make people unique, right? Even the most admired celebrities and A-listers have flaws – often airbrushed out of the images you see of them. Your imperfections might not even be as bad as you make them out to be but whatever they are, they are a part of you. Own them, embrace them, and stop worrying about them.

Reassess your core beliefs. You might not like second-guessing your beliefs because they are what keep you going. But if they are destructive or undermining your potential, you need to rethink them. Many of them will be based on what others have told you about yourself in the past, and some of them will be your own way of protecting yourself from pain or upset.

When you have low self-esteem, you might be following rules that are just not right, such as always wanting to please people, or avoiding the risk of criticism. You need to have a long, hard think about which beliefs are harming you and get rid of them.

Recovering from low self esteem doesn't happen overnight but it is possible with time. Once you begin to implement some of the changes I've mentioned above, you will feel more powerful, in control, and happier about yourself.

Take back your power and start living your life, regardless of what anyone says or does!

Highlights

- **Self-esteem is the opinion you have of yourself and low self-esteem can make your life miserable.**
- **Only you can increase your positive feelings about who you are and what you are capable of.**

- **Low self-esteem affects every aspect of your life, from your relationships to your physical and mental health.**
- **The way you think of yourself often comes from how others treated you.**
- **Negative self-talk also fills your mind full of self-doubt and low confidence.**
- **Bad habits reinforce your lack of self-esteem but you can change them.**
- **By believing in yourself and reassessing your core values, you can rise up and enjoy a truly fulfilling life on your own terms.**

6
THE 7 TOP TURN ONS IN MEN

"*A man cannot be comfortable without his own approval.*" – Mark Twain

Darren is a young entrepreneur in his late 20s who I have been coaching for a while now. On his recent visit, he filled me in about his plans for expanding his tech start-up business before we got chatting about his personal life.

He told me how frustrated he feels because although he is good-looking, financially sound, has his own place, and a snazzy sports car to boot, he can't seem to find a girlfriend. To his mind, he had everything a woman could want but found himself being rejected by them time after time.

Although Darren is a lovely guy, I could see where he was going wrong. He had this idea that physical good looks, money, and status are enough to hook a girlfriend. It seems natural to assume that, especially nowadays when there is so much emphasis on our appearance and how well we are doing in life.

I think that many men, Darren included, haven't stopped to think that there is more to attraction than that. In fact, all the research shows that the laws of attraction are very subtle and have more to do with non-verbal behavior than you may think.

If you are feeling the same way as Darren and wondering why your dating life is almost non-existent, you need to read this chapter. Of course, looks do play their part in attracting someone's attention, but they really aren't everything. I know plenty of women who are attracted to men you wouldn't typically describe as handsome, athletic, wealthy, or 'a good catch'.

You probably do too, and have often asked yourself, 'What does she see in him?' Well, the answer to that is, 'She sees the real him, and finds that attractive.' Outward appearances and status symbols might dazzle a few people but when it comes to real attraction that could lead to a long-term partnership, that's a different thing altogether.

At the end of the day, it seems to come down to a few essentials, like how confident you are in yourself and how you convey this to others.

Now, if you aren't feeling particularly confident at the moment, that can sound like bad news. Your low self-esteem and negativity might be so overpowering that your chances of ever finding a girlfriend seem to be fading into the distance as we speak.

The thing is, you can learn to be confident and a lot of this book is dedicated to just that. After all, when you begin to love yourself, that will be obvious to anyone you meet. Self-confidence is something you build over time and you will get there eventually, trust me.

Why does confidence matter?

There's nothing more potent than confidence but I don't mean the cocky kind where you act as if you are God's gift to women. I'm talking about the inner confidence that comes through knowing who you are and being 'your own man'. No matter how many material trophies you have in your life, they aren't much good if you use them to cover up your insecurities and self-doubts.

A truly confident man doesn't need any of those things. Sure, they are nice to have, and can even build up your ego and make you feel good, but they are no substitute for authentic confidence.

In the same way, not having the flash car, cool clothes, or Brad Pitt looks doesn't stop you from attracting women. As I said, the way you behave and interact is much more likely to bring you success.

You don't need to be wealthy, a top-league soccer player or six-foot-tall to woo women. You just have to be yourself, minus the insecurities and lack of self-esteem. Most women are attracted to men who feel good about themselves and everything else is secondary to that.

Fighting your fears

Having the confidence to strike up a conversation with a woman in the first place is a daunting task for many men. The idea of going over to talk to someone you like, especially someone you don't know, might be a terrifying thought. What if she rejects you, isn't interested in you, or even laughs in your face?

Fear of being rejected is a great way to never meet anyone in your life. It's guaranteed to protect you from being hurt or humiliated, but it is also going to stop you from finding a girlfriend or partner. Bad experiences in your past might have left you feeling hurt and your self-protection mode is always activated.

That is totally understandable because it's a natural survival response after all, with that old saying, 'once bitten, twice shy' making a lot of sense.

When you are in this survival mindset, fear serves a purpose – to keep you alive and well. The last thing your brain is thinking about is romance, sex, and courtship. What you need to do is shift gears and tell yourself the fear you are feeling isn't serving any purpose anymore.

Your past rejection has no bearing on whether or not you will be rejected again and hanging on to that misconception is only blocking you from meeting someone new.

Expecting the worst

If thoughts run through your head like, 'She won't be interested in me, she's far too good for me,' then that says more about how you view yourself than how anyone else sees you. This comes down to your low self-esteem, which is preventing you from believing that anyone would want to be with you.

A man who is self-assured doesn't worry about this as he knows his own worth and value. If he wants to approach a woman, he doesn't torture himself about whether it will go well or not. And if the woman he talks to isn't interested in him, he doesn't take it to heart. He is confident enough to take the rejection without internalizing it as a criticism of who he is.

Letting go of expectations is truly liberating because it allows you to take action without being stressed about how things will develop. If you are planning to have a night out and socialize, think of it as an adventure instead of a mating mission. You might seriously want to meet someone but that just takes the joy out of having a good time with friends and being relaxed. Rather than thinking about what you will do or say if you see the woman (or man) of your dreams across the room, focus on looking forward to a chilled night out where anything could happen.

When you set more realistic expectations, you are less likely to go home feeling miserable because you didn't meet anyone. It is fine to tell yourself that tonight could be the night and to get excited about that prospect, but don't make it the only reason to go out.

Stay open to possibilities by all means, because you never know what could happen, but avoid building your hopes up every single time you hit the town. That will often leave you feeling disappointed and unlovable.

If you can manage to overcome your fear and have some kind of conversation starter prepared beforehand, this will help you to get off to a good start. I'll be giving you some examples later on in this chapter that you can use when you want to talk to someone. They will help you to break the ice and have something to say instead of feeling nervous and tongue-tied.

Would you date yourself?

If your answer to the above question is no, why is that? Obviously, you know your flaws but are they so bad that they make you undateable? Most women have a kind of radar that tells them when a man feels unhappy about himself and any negativity is easily detected. Self-love shows, so it's important to nurture it, otherwise, how can you expect anyone else to love you?

If you are full of self-loathing, tend to play the victim, and don't radiate positive vibes from within, that acts as a repellent. On the other hand, when you take pride in your appearance, pursue your passions, and show self-respect, this is like catnip to most women.

Think about the following statements and choose any that resonate with you. This will give you a good idea of how 'attractive' you may appear to a potential partner even before you begin talking to them:

1. I am a man who goes after what he wants
2. I respect my physical and emotional wellbeing
3. I invest time pursuing my passions
4. I take pride in my appearance
5. I stay true to my core values

NONE of the above are written on your forehead, although the way you behave, talk, and interact with others makes them very evident. Of course, your outward appearance is the first thing that people notice but after that, there are a whole lot of other things going on that make you 'attractive' to someone else.

Imagine that you see a gorgeous woman across the room and find her incredibly attractive from a physical standpoint. The way she moves, laughs, and acts will then either increase or decrease the attraction you feel for her. If, for example, she smokes, that might be a big turn-off for you.

What if she laughs too loudly or is sitting with hunched shoulders looking miserable? Do you go over and talk to her or get put off by how she is behaving?

Let's say that you do decide to approach her and she leans in too close to you, invading your personal space, or seems nervous and bites her nails when you try to speak to her.

What is her behavior telling you about how comfortable she is? Now, imagine a woman approaching you and you act in the same way as above. How attractive do you think that will be to her? In other words, attraction is about more than just the physical aspect of ourselves.

Are you sexually attractive?

You might wonder if anyone could find you remotely attractive but sexual attraction is a funny thing that we don't have much control over. It is regulated by the limbic system – a primitive part of the brain that controls our essential functions.

When you meet a potential mate, your hypothalamus releases chemicals like dopamine and serotonin that generate feelings of lust or love. By the same token, anyone who finds you sexually attractive will have the same biological reaction.

In her book, *Love Demystified,* Professor Palmer of California State University notes that we tend to be drawn to people who are similar to us or who remind us of loved ones. Our hormones are activated subconsciously when the other person triggers a kind of resemblance to someone we know.

Smell also plays an important role (I can't stress enough the power of a good deodorant!) in the attraction game, with certain odors turning people on or off.

Who we consider to be good-looking is mainly a cultural thing, which makes sense. Attractive physical features are closely related to how healthy, youthful, and fertile we think someone is, and depending on where we live, there are a wide variety of norms.

Whether you like a classic voluptuous figure or find the slim body type appealing, these preferences are usually bound up with trends about what society thinks is beautiful. Living in the western world, you probably know that the current 'ideal build' for a man is reasonably muscular, healthy-looking, and around 172 cm tall (5ft 8 in).

Not fitting into that stereotype might make you feel unattractive and undesirable, although it's important to understand that there are plenty of guys fitting that description who also have trouble finding a partner. Let me remind you again – looks aren't everything!

What personal qualities are attractive?

There are a lot of other qualities women look for in a potential partner, with some general traits that we all find appealing. As you read the points below, I want you to consider which aspects you could work on to improve your chances of attracting women. This list is by no means exhaustive, but it will give you some idea of what matters in the dating game.

- **Being comfortable in yourself**

If you're not happy with who you are, it is difficult to convince someone else that they should be with you. Do you know what your best attributes are and show them whenever you meet someone new or do you emphasize your flaws? No one is going to find you attractive if you talk about all of your bad points – it is a real turn-off.

- **Being able to laugh at yourself**

If you take yourself too seriously, that can be off-putting for many people. The ability to make the occasional joke about something you did is very endearing as it shows you accept you aren't perfect.

On the other hand, making yourself look like an absolute fool is not that appealing. Being able to laugh at yourself, and make others laugh too, requires a bit of skill but can raise your attraction level if done with confidence.[1]

- **Being happy with your looks**

Whatever your body type and fitness level, they shouldn't get in the way of how you feel about yourself. If you do think you need to lose some weight or want to sculpt those muscles, by all means, go for it.

Following a healthy diet and maintaining a regular workout routine will definitely boost your confidence but you don't have to be a bodybuilder to be attractive. It's how you feel about your body that counts.

Dressing well, keeping your clothes clean, and making the effort to look nice will do wonders for your self-esteem, too.

- **Being in love with life**

If you want to be attractive, having a positive outlook on life acts like a magnet. Being unhappy with your job, studies, or social standing can be a big put off, because that discontentment comes across when you interact with others.

No one wants to hear a potential partner moaning about their miserable life, but talking about your goals to improve your situation and achieve something better is alluring.

- **Being passionate about your interests and hobbies**

When you are passionate about activities or interests, others will find you interesting – the kind of guy they want to learn more about. If you don't feel passionate about anything, think about what you enjoy doing – it could be a sport or a creative pursuit – and start spending more time doing it. As long as you aren't obsessive about it, having a passion is a very appealing quality.

- **Being curious**

If you are interested in new people, places, and cultures, not only do you get a different perspective on life but you also have more to talk about. Rather than making boring conversation, you can impress with your knowledge and ability to talk about a variety of topics, which make you great to be around.

- **Being on good terms with others**

When you get on well with your family and friends, this shows you appreciate your loved ones. No one wants to meet a guy who finds it hard to maintain good relationships with his relatives because this might show he doesn't get on with people or can't build close bonds. If you feel that this describes you, it might be time to consider how you can establish better ties with your family and deepen your existing friendships. That doesn't mean you have to accept toxic relationships or continue to mix with people who disrespect you. It is more about paying attention to those you value and spending more time with them.

The 7 top turn-ons

The above are all general qualities that anyone should pay attention to but when it comes to more manly traits, there are a few additional things that seem to attract women. Although gender equality has leveled out the playing field in areas like financial independence, career choices, and sexual liberation, women generally still look for the following **7 top turn-ons** in men:

1. You know how to lead.

Whether it be as a dance partner or a travel buddy, women want to feel like they are with a leader: someone they can trust and rely on. That doesn't mean being a tyrant and always having your way or controlling her. A good leader always considers the impact of their decisions on others, puts their needs at the forefront, and initiates activities to nourish the relationship.

2. You know how to listen.

When a woman talks, it is important to be a good listener and not talk over her, otherwise, she will feel disrespected by you. That means listening without interrupting but knowing when to add the occasional, 'I understand how you feel...' You don't always have to provide the answers to all her problems either – simply allowing her to express how she feels and showing empathy is often all it takes.

3. You know how to communicate.

The things you talk about can make you extremely appealing. Being able to express your goals, ambitions, fears, beliefs, and values allows the other person to get to know you and this helps to form strong bonds.

In fact, women enjoy discovering that you are sensitive, thoughtful, and willing to open up about your feelings so don't hold back. Spend an equal amount of time talking and listening if you want to create a dialogue that could advance to something more meaningful.

4. You know how to care.

Thinking about the needs of others and behaving selflessly are qualities that women truly appreciate. For example, being willing to sacrifice a night out with your buddies to check in on a sick relative will score you a lot of points in a female's eyes.

Showing compassion toward those worse off than yourself, caring about animal welfare, and putting your beliefs into action are all highly-regarded traits that make you more attractive than you can imagine.

5. You practice mindfulness.

This might sound like a weird one, but a study carried out in Australia in 2015 found that men practicing mindfulness tend to rate higher on the attractiveness scale.[2]

Mindful statements made by the male participants of the study were shown to attract a greater number of women than statements that weren't of a similar nature, proving that the more you are in tune with yourself, the cuter you are! The kind of things a person who practices mindfulness would say that are taken from the study include:

– I perceive my feelings and emotions without having to react to them.

– I notice changes in my body, such as whether my breathing slows down or speeds up.

– I'm good at finding the words to describe my feelings.

6. You smell good!

Although you might think that women are turned on by the odor of macho sweat, the truth is that this only applies when the sweat is fresh. That's when a chemical called androstenol is produced. Once it begins to oxidize, this smell becomes a complete turn-off for women so if you can't produce fresh sweat on demand, using deodorant is a must.

Another study has shown that the use of colognes and aftershave also improves your mood, making you behave more confidently.[3] This helps to attract more potential partners even though it is you that is drawing them in with your positive energy and not related to the smell of the cologne itself.

7. You use body language

Non-verbal behavior can have a strong influence on how attractive women find you. There's nothing like a man standing tall with his chest out and his head held high to signal confidence and this is something you can easily do.

Smiling is also a big plus in your favor – no one finds grumpy people appealing or fun to be around so flash those teeth as often as you can. When it comes to flirting, an observational study carried out by Life-Labs Learning in 2004[4] showed that men who were successful with women displayed specific kinds of certain kinds of non-verbal behavior such as:

- More short-term glancing at women to signal sexual interest through eye contact
- More movements to take up space and assert dominance, such as moving your arms and legs about.
- Touching other men more in a non-sexual way as a sign of authority or dominance.
- Less closed-body movements such as folding your arms or crossing your legs.

BONUS TIP – Keep yourself well-groomed

Fads in facial and body hair may come and go but all the surveys done by leading magazines like Men's Health and GQ reveal that being well-groomed will definitely make you more attractive.

No matter what look you are going for – trendy fashionista, street style guy, or rugged rock star – taking care of your appearance matters. From the hair on your head right down to your little toenails, looking after yourself shows you value yourself, and others will appreciate that too. Pay particular attention to the following:

- **Get a proper haircut**

No matter what hairstyle you prefer, make sure you visit your barber regularly to keep it looking good. Even if you like long hair, a regular trim can keep it sharp. If you can afford it, invest in a multi-purpose trimmer to freshen up your haircut, as well as your sideburns and neck. Don't forget to trim your eyebrows too if they are too long or bushy.

- **Style your hair**

There are now thousands of hair styling products on the market for men, so don't be afraid to try some of them. You only need to use a tiny bit of hair gel to get your hair under control and if you are feeling creative, you can sculpt it, slick it back, tie it, straighten it, or curl it. Let your inner man come through and make heads turn!

- **Look after your facial hair**

Whether you like showing a bit of a 5 o'clock shadow or prefer to sport a full-grown beard, it seems that women like facial hair on men. Beards can be a fashion statement and also represent status or maturity, depending on the culture.

A study carried out in the UK in 2008 found that the women taking part viewed males with a full beard as the most masculine, men with a light beard as the most dominant, and those with light stubble the most attractive.[5]

For that reason, make sure whatever facial hair you grow always looks clean and trim. Keep it tidy by using one of the beard balms, oils, and beard brushes on the market and make a good impression with the opposite sex.

- **Take care of your teeth.**

Bad teeth are not appealing and, apart from that, can seriously damage your confidence. Most people with dental issues like crooked teeth, missing teeth, or yellow teeth, are embarrassed about that and will try to hide it in public. That may mean trying not to smile, or covering your mouth with your hand when you laugh, both of which simply draw attention to the fact that you have a problem.

A smile can win over hearts and minds, as well as attract women so don't neglect your dentures or your oral hygiene (and that includes bad breath).

Visit a dentist every six months and have your teeth cleaned professionally to remove any plaque. Get into the habit of brushing your teeth twice a day – it only takes a few minutes each time – and use a breath freshener before you go out. If you do need dental work, put it on your list of priorities so you can eventually achieve that perfect winning smile.

The whole point of taking care of your looks is to make you feel more confident. Whichever style of dress, haircut, and facial/body hair you prefer, take pride in your overall appearance every day because it is the first thing others will notice about you.

You want to give yourself the best chance possible of creating a good first impression and when you feel good about yourself, you will be hard to resist!

Highlights

- **Physical good looks, money, and status are not enough to attract a girlfriend.**

- Inner confidence and being 'your own man' can be more appealing than flashy cars.
- Fear of possible rejection or expecting the worst outcome can prevent you from ever finding a future partner.
- If you wouldn't date yourself, you can't expect anyone else to want to date you.
- Not fitting into the cultural stereotype of what an attractive man should look like might seriously affect your confidence.
- Women look for a range of inner qualities in men, such as passion, curiosity, positivity, humor, and compassion.
- Showing leadership, the ability to communicate, practicing mindfulness, smelling good, and using positive body language are all attractive traits you can learn.
- Being well-groomed, clean, and tidy is a definite turn-on for women.

7
ARE YOU HELPING OR HURTING OTHERS?

"Remember that the happiest people are not those getting more, but those giving more." –Robin Sharma

Kindness is a moral virtue most of us have grown up learning about. From little kids, we are told to be kind, help those in need, and the importance of giving rather than receiving. The problem is that life might have treated you so badly that you find it hard to stretch out a helping hand to anyone.

When you feel unloved, under-appreciated, or have a hard time loving yourself, it can be hard to spread kindness to those around you. Painful past experiences could make you mistrust people and not want to offer to help anyone.

Even though you aren't a bad person, you might not feel that you have anything to offer anyone in the way of help. You might also purposefully avoid going out of your way to be helpful because no one ever helps you.

There are other reasons why you may not be too keen to help others: perhaps you are worried about offending someone or that your actions will be misinterpreted. Should you give up your seat on the train for the woman standing next to you or will you get a barrage of insults because you are implying she is inferior to you?

A thought like that could stop you from carrying out a simple act of kindness in whatever context.

You might have a fear of talking to strangers or think that being kind is a sign of weakness. In this age of toxic masculinity, you certainly don't want to be accused of being a wimp and that could affect how willing you are to help others. I can see how that might make you think it's easier to keep to yourself than to offer a helping hand to anyone who needs it, although you aren't doing yourself any favors if this is the case.

All the science shows that there are many benefits to helping others, such as improving your overall health, experiencing less stress, and boosting your energy levels. Being kind to others can make you feel more connected to them and even happier in yourself. In reality, kindness is a strength, not a weakness, and any time you help someone, you are boosting your self-esteem and well-being.

What can kindness bring you?

Research provides compelling data on the benefits of helping others through the use of MRI technology. Basically, this kind of testing measures brain activity in relation to changes in blood flow and neural activity.

As a result, we now know that giving activates the same parts of the brain that are stimulated by food and sex. In other words, being kind or helpful is a pleasurable experience! It could even be the secret to living a healthier, happier life that is filled with more meaning and purpose.

If you can remember the last time someone helped you, you will know how nice that feels. Simple things like a kind word, someone helping you carry a heavy item up some steps, or receiving a small gift – all of these can change how you feel about yourself. The act of giving can also have the same effect and it doesn't have to be a grand gesture or involve giving away large sums of money.

It is the act itself that leaves you feeling good, and not the scale of it or the cost. A simple 'thank you' from someone you have helped can really make you feel good inside and improve your self-worth and confidence so why not give it a shot?

Helping others without having anything to gain from that is known as altruism. It's the good deeds people do every day without expecting anything in return.

Helping someone to cross the road, looking in on an elderly neighbor, or offering to help a colleague out at work are all acts of altruism. The reward you get is knowing you have made a small but meaningful impact on someone's life and that's a win-win situation. There is nothing better than the sense of pride you can enjoy afterward and once you start, you will find it becomes a lot easier to do in the future.

Now is a good time to think about what random acts of kindness you could do today, or tomorrow. You could note a couple of things or you could promise yourself to help at least one person every day. It can be anything you feel comfortable with, such as:

- Putting a few coins in the tin of the homeless guy you pass every day
- Making a special breakfast for your partner, parents, or housemate
- Offering to take a neighbor's dog for a walk
- Buying a coffee for a colleague who is having a bad day
- Giving up your seat on the bus for a senior citizen

When you think about it, there are so many things you can do in just 24 hours to make a difference in someone else's life. And remember that the more kind acts you do, the better you will feel, too.

An article published in the National Library of Medicine in 2016[1] described a study in which members of the public were asked to either perform acts of kindness for one month or to perform kind acts for themselves, like treating themselves to a new purchase.

When the participants' level of 'psychological flourishing' was measured (that is, their emotional, psychological, and social well-being) at the start and end of the study, the results were clear. Those who had carried out kind acts for others reported a higher degree of positive emotions than those who just treated themselves.

A natural high

Those uplifting feelings can also benefit your physical well-being in four key ways:

Being kind releases feel-good hormones

Performing kind acts for others releases serotonin in your brain, which is the feel-good hormone. Your endorphin levels also rise, leading to what is often called a 'helper's high' – similar to a high that a mild dose of morphine can give you.

Being kind reduces anxiety

If you suffer from social anxiety, you will probably find it difficult to experience positive moods like joy, interest, and alertness. Acting in a kind manner can reduce that anxiety because you suddenly feel relevant and capable of achieving something in your life. It is a very empowering feeling and one that can eventually help you to lead a more fulfilling life with less anxiety.

Kindness might help to overcome certain illnesses

There is a mountain of evidence to suggest that inflammation in the body is linked to certain health problems, like chronic pain, migraines, obesity, and diabetes. The older you get, the more susceptible you are to such conditions but you can heal yourself by volunteering.

One study published in The Gerontologist in 2014[2] showed that adults in the age range of 57-85 who regularly volunteered (in their local community, for example) had lower levels of inflammation than those who didn't. The oxytocin that is released when you are kind also has a positive impact on the health of your heart, with the nitric oxide it produces helping to dilate the blood vessels and reduce blood pressure.

That's a great reason to do good to others and look after your health at the same time!

Kindness reduces stress

When you are caught up in your own problems, they often become magnified and can cause you to feel in a constant state of stress. By helping others, you are taking your mind off whatever is worrying you and forget your own issues for a little while. As well as that, the more interaction you have with others, the more social bonds you can develop and fewer feelings of isolation.

Unlike antisocial behavior, prosocial behavior can alleviate stress and allow you to deal with it better, therefore reducing its negative impact on you. Who knows – by connecting with others you might even establish a life-long friendship or find the love of your life, and that is definitely something worth having!

How to help yourself by helping others

Instead of being wrapped up in your own life, with all its problems, there are many ways you can help others that don't require hard labor or large chunks of your time.

You can do your bit every day, or even take on a long-term commitment to help others in a specific way. Knowing now what the benefits of helping are to yourself and those you help out, there is nothing to stop you!

One thing to bear in mind is that you shouldn't offer to help to the point that you are depleted of your energy. If your actions are exhausting physically or mentally, you might be doing too much. Kindness begins with yourself so don't overdo it and neglect your own needs.

It's important to also maintain your boundaries and to say 'no' to helping out if you feel it is encroaching on your comfort zone. Do what you can, when you can, and with a happy heart rather than a begrudging one.

Here are a few ways you can extend a helping hand and begin to enjoy that feeling of worthiness, value, and fulfillment:

Volunteering

This is a great way to help others and increase your levels of self-esteem and well-being. You will find many local charities and community organizations only too happy to welcome you so check out which ones you are interested in before approaching them.

- Maybe help out at your local youth club, where you can pass on some of your skills or offer to be a mentor.
- Offer to help out at a local library or somewhere you know they are probably understaffed.
- Hospitals often need volunteers to keep patients company, read them stories, and so on, which you may be interested in doing.

Helping out a good cause

You might want to help the environment, reduce poverty, or stop animal cruelty, all of which you can do if you put some time and energy into it. Any cause that is close to your heart is worth pursuing and your involvement in that will give you a wonderful sense of achievement.

- You can support the cause financially – every little helps.
- Support them on social media and sign up for their newsletter so you can keep up to date with their activities.
- Help them to organize a fund-raising event or take part in a sponsored mini-marathon to raise money.

Small acts of kindness

If you do not feel inspired to volunteer or help a good cause, you can still carry out small acts of kindness with people you know. Whether they are family members, friends, colleagues, or neighbors, they will appreciate any help they receive from you and kind gestures so feel free to spread the love.

Call a friend or sibling you haven't spoken to for a while

Ask your neighbor if they want any help with the gardening or shopping

Help out more with household chores if you live with others

Write a 'thank you' note to someone who was kind to you recently

Check in on someone you know who is going through a difficult period at the moment

Say good morning or 'hello' to people you see every day – you will be amazed at how good that feels for them and yourself.

Volunteer to help someone when they are having difficulty with something you are good at.

Be willing to listen to someone's problems without judgment or criticism.

Be a considerate driver and allow others to have priority (if the highway code permits that).

Pick up any trash lying around in the street, public park, or beach.

Be nice on social media and resist the urge to leave insulting, offensive comments when you see something you don't agree with or dislike.

Reach out to people you know who seem to be going through a tough time, telling them you are sorry to hear about whatever has happened.

Instead of getting caught up in rumors, unsubstantiated stories, or hate speech, be compassionate and show your support for the rights of others.

How much compassion do you have?

Although compassion is generally seen by society as a feminine trait, it is in fact a strength that all men are capable of too. It is compassion that makes you courageous, even heroic, whether by rescuing a kitten from a tree or saving someone from drowning.

Despite cultural stereotypes of how men should be tough, it's images of men helping out their friends, family, colleagues, and peers that convey more strength than anything else.

According to Dr. Ted Zeff, author of *Raise an Emotionally Healthy Boy*, only compassionate men can save the planet, but not the aggressive, unemotional type. It's the kind, loving man, who is brave enough to be gentle and compassionate – something many men have a knee-jerk reaction to because it goes against traditional views of masculinity. If you can peel away that armor, it will be easier for you to connect with others in a more meaningful way and be able to express the whole spectrum of your emotions.

You can begin by exercising some self-compassion, which is a great way to nourish your inner wellbeing. When you can do that, it will be easier for you to reach out to others with more empathy and understanding. Here are my essential tips to help you begin the process:

Treat yourself as you would treat a friend. How do you respond when a close friend is struggling and what kind of things do you tell them to help them? Now, think about the times when you feel down – how do you respond to yourself? If you notice any difference between the two, why is that? How would you feel if you started treating yourself like a friend?

Give yourself a break. If you are under a lot of stress or facing problems in your life, how are you dealing with it? Can you acknowledge that you are suffering, in pain, or feeling hurt? Tell yourself that others also experience this kind of pain and that you are not alone. You are allowed to be compassionate with yourself and to accept your emotions as legitimate. Be strong, be patient, and be kind to your inner self whenever you are struggling to cope.

Identify what you really want. Do you use self-criticism as a motivator and come down hard on yourself in the hope that will make you change?

Judging yourself harshly will only generate more self-loathing, so instead of doing that, try to get to the source of the pain your self-criticism is causing you. Exercise self-compassion and find a healthier way to motivate yourself that includes positive encouragement and kindness.

Your well-being comes before anything else so allow for a bit of 'me time' without guilt. Allocate a part of your day to relaxing and reflecting on how you are doing.

Spend time away from social media and treat yourself to something small, like a new haircut or the latest video game. Indulge in your passions: cook, dance, paint, go for a walk, play with the dog, or whatever brings you joy and happiness.

If you really want to be kinder to others you need to begin practicing self-kindness first. Self-love not only empowers you to be stronger, but it also allows you to be more compassionate to others, and that is true strength!

Highlights

- **Kindness is a strength, not a weakness.**
- **The brain is stimulated by being kind and helpful in the same way it experiences the pleasure of food and sex.**
- **One good deed a day keeps the doctor away.**
- **Being kind reduces stress, anxiety, and inflammation, and provides a natural high.**
- **When you help others, you help yourself.**
- **Volunteering or helping out a good cause will increase your well-being.**
- **Small acts of kindness make the world a much better place.**
- **Practice self-compassion so you can show compassion to others.**

8
IT'S TIME TO PUT IT ALL INTO PRACTICE

"A man's got to have a code, a creed to live by, no matter his job."
–John Wayne

If you are still struggling to accept the term 'self-love' as a masculine thing, that is understandable. You have probably been brought up in a culture where the idea of what it is to be a real man is slightly warped. Music, movies, video games, and social media have been pumping out distorted ideas about how men should behave for decades, so it's no wonder that you may be a bit hesitant.

After all, you don't want to be called a soft touch, a momma's boy, or accused of having no balls.

These kinds of name-calling reactions usually come from men who are also afraid to be called the same, or from women who have also bought into the 'man in a box' culture.

But none of that should stop you from forging your own path in life and being the man you want to be. To be honest, there has never been a better time to be a man and that's because you can now show your emotions, be gentle, stay at home to look after the kids, and enjoy doing things once limited to the female domain.

You should celebrate that fact because it's only when you live in line with your true self that you can really enjoy life to the full.

There is no need to follow trends, succumb to peer pressure, or play a role that just doesn't represent you anymore. You CAN be the man you want to be and still earn respect from those around you. You can be nurturing, protective, brave, strong, and lead all at the same time. It doesn't have to be an either/or scenario anymore where you need to either act like a caveman or be a soppy wimp.

You can be both tough and tender, rough and romantic, strong and sensitive – you can be all you want to be.

Society versus biology

Masculinity generally describes the social expectations of what it is to be a man and refers to certain roles, behaviors, and attributes. To that extent, masculinity is a social construct backed by certain historical and political trends, rather than having anything to do with biology.

Maleness, on the other hand, refers to the anatomical and physiological characteristics of being male. It involves *the feelings and experiences of being male as a result of an XY chromosomal orientation.*[1] It's disturbing to think that so much of maleness and masculinity (and femininity) depends on your genitals or social conditioning when clearly, we are all more than that.

This chapter is dedicated to giving you the space to explore your inner self and to create your own definition of what it means to be you, and what kind of man you wish to be.

You can begin by answering the following ten questions, which are aimed at helping you to appraise the personal beliefs you have about yourself. They will get you to think about how positively you see yourself, and how critical you are about your perceived flaws. Take some time to think about each one before you answer as honestly as you can, without worrying if you are right or wrong.

1. What is your favorite thing about yourself? Why?
2. What are your most achievable goals in life?

3. How do you handle criticism?
4. What past accomplishments are you proud of?
5. How do you feel when you make a mistake? What do you do?
6. How do you feel when someone compliments you?
7. What do you feel you are really good at?
8. If you could do anything with your life right now, what would it be?
9. What makes you feel good about yourself?
10. When do you feel most comfortable 'being yourself'?

Once you become more aware of your personal beliefs about yourself, you can begin to understand the influence that they have over you.

At that point, it will be easier for you to replace any negative beliefs with positive ones and become more accepting of who you are.

This leads to more self-love and allows you to grow into a happier, more balanced man.

Self-love in practice

The main problem you might have with self-love is that you simply don't like yourself. This is a habit you need to break because it is stopping you from getting the most out of life.

It takes time to change these negative thought patterns but you can rewire the system by introducing new habits into your life.

To help you do that, I want you to think about the different dimensions of yourself, which can be divided into 4 main categories: the **physical, mental, emotional, and spiritual**. Let's take a look at each one and discover how you can nurture more self-love every day:

1. Physical self-love

Get enough sleep, which is crucial for your physical and mental health. Instead of sitting up late to watch TV or stream a movie on your laptop, go to bed at a regular time each night. Depending on your work schedule and lifestyle, that could be 9 pm or 12 midnight - the point is to make sure you get ample sleep because you need it.

Eat healthily as often as you can, which basically means incorporating fresh food into your diet and removing processed foods. If you can't live without fast food or pizza, limit these to once a week and for the other days, eat plenty of vegetables, fruit, wholegrain foods, and high-protein foods for energy.

Exercise regularly to keep your joints and muscles in good working order, as well as your heart. Ideally, you should get about 150 minutes of moderate aerobic activity or 75 minutes of vigorous aerobic activity each week. If you like lifting weights, try some skipping exercises too and if you are into sports, join one of your local teams. Walk, run, swim, and let your body know you care about it.

Look after your personal hygiene to avoid any unnecessary health problems such as skin, teeth, or hair & nail problems. Establish a daily grooming ritual that includes having a bath or shower, brushing your teeth twice a day, using dental floss, applying skin moisturizer, and keeping your nails short and manicured.

Drink plenty of water and nutritious beverages. Water is important for our overall physical performance and the good news is you can drink as much of it as you like. You should be drinking at least 3-4 liters per day and if your tap water isn't good quality, use a filter or buy bottled water.

Tea is well known for its wellness benefits and there is a whole range of different flavors you can try out, depending on your tastes. Fresh fruit juice is also packed with essential nutrients and if you have a blender, you can also make smoothies.

Combine the fruit of your liking with veggies such as carrots and flavorings like ginger to put a spring in your step each morning.

Get out more and reconnect with nature, be that at a local park, in the mountains, by a lake, on a beach, or in a forest. If you don't want to go it alone, join a local hiking or climbing club, which will probably organize weekly events that you can join. You will even get to socialize and make some new friends, which is a wonderful thing in itself!

Go for a massage once a month and enjoy the physical sensation of being touched in a non-sexual manner. Not only will it do your body the world of good, but it will also relax and de-stress you. Otherwise, ask for a hug from your loved ones now and again or offer to give them one when you see them. You could even get a pet if you feel you can look after it and just having something to stroke or hold can have a wonderful calming effect, as well as provide you with company.

2. Mental self-love

Your brain needs stimulation but be careful about what kind of things you feed it. It is much healthier to read a good book than to waste your time reading social media posts. Reading for just half an hour each day is a great way to take your mind off your problems and escape. It also helps to improve your vocabulary and your perceptions of the world, opening your mind up to new possibilities and interests.

Try doing some crossword puzzles or sudoku to keep your brain on its toes. There are lots of free apps available to download onto your smartphone so that you can do puzzles with words or numbers wherever you are.

Whichever you prefer, this is a great way to get your gray matter working and exercise your cognitive abilities.

Practice meditation, which is an ancient technique used to help reduce stress and improve self-awareness. It only takes a few minutes each day and the more you practice, the better you will become.

There are hundreds of easy-to-follow meditation videos on Youtube for beginners so check them out and find a channel that you like. Before you know it, you will be wondering how you managed to live without meditation in your life!

3. Emotional self-love

It's very important to tend to your emotional side, even though this may be the most difficult thing for you to do. Past traumas, social conditioning, and painful experiences may have left you feeling unable to explore your emotions, preferring to bury them under a very thick skin.

Begin by simply being grateful for one small thing in your life before you go to sleep each night. You could give thanks for being alive, healthy, and for having a roof over your head.

As you get used to giving gratitude, you can make a list of five things you are grateful for in your life each week and just by writing them down, you are learning how to heal emotionally.

Find a way to express yourself. When you can put feelings into words, you reduce the power they have over you and can feel more emotionally balanced.

Get into the habit of writing down those feelings in a notebook or journal and then reading out loud what you have written. This will help you to see them from a different perspective and feel released from any stress or anxiety you were carrying around with you.

4. Spiritual self-love

You do not need to be religious to practice spiritual self-love and can still take care of your spiritual needs even if you have never set foot in a church or temple. Meditation is one way to get in touch with your inner self and prayer can also serve that purpose.

Any activity that allows you to tap into your essence and reflect on your being can alleviate negative feelings such as anger and nurture positive emotions like compassion.

Knowing that you are more than just a body can be a transformative experience that brings you greater wisdom and healing so dedicate some time each day to this important aspect of yourself.

Learn more about your own religion and get involved with your local church if you feel the need. It could allow you to meet with like-minded people and establish new bonds with others.

Learn more about the belief systems of others and take any wisdom from them if you find something you align with. There are so many ways in which people express their beliefs and you might discover new ideas that resonate with you at a spiritual level. Nourish your inner needs and develop a stronger sense of self-love as you journey along your spiritual path.

Declaring self-love

By now, you should be able to recognize where you have been neglecting yourself, and ways to cultivate more self-love. If you are not into journaling but would like to write down the ways in which you feel you have improved, I am providing you with a few sentences you can fill in.

Hopefully, you will find this easier to do than before you began reading this book. Once you get into the habit of making this kind of self-assessment, you will be inspired by how far you have come and motivated to keep working on self-love.

If you can't complete all of the sentences, keep coming back to them at regular intervals to see if anything has changed that will allow you to fill them in.

The three things I love best about myself are i .... ii .... and iii ....

.... is something I want to cultivate in my life.

This week, I'm going to reward myself by ....

I've decided not to worry about ....

Someone recently told me I have great ....

I deserve to feel good because I ....

.... is something that others admire about me.

I'm so looking forward to ....

I am proud to have achieved ....

I can't change .... and I choose to accept it.

I get better at ....every day.

I feel happy because I ....

Today, I feel great because I managed to ……………

One thing I love about me is that I ……………

This week, I'm giving myself a break from thinking about …………

You are worthy of self-love

Everyone deserves to love themselves, no matter what their imperfections or flaws are. No one is perfect, after all, but that doesn't stop us from being worthy of a fulfilling, happy life. The only way to feel better about yourself is by truly believing that you matter and working toward your end goal.

It's important to get away from this idea of perfection, which seems to make even the most accomplished person feel like a failure. There is no such thing as a perfect dad, brother, husband, friend, or partner. If that were the case, life would be extremely dull.

You can start by acknowledging your weaknesses and stop torturing yourself over every little mistake you make. Failing to achieve something or not being Mr. Perfect does not mean you should be excluded from enjoying love and connection with others. Happiness is a human right that was even written into a United Nations resolution in 2012 on the International Day of Happiness.[2]

As the K-Pop band BTS said in their award-winning song entitled Love Yourself, it's more difficult to love ourselves than to love somebody else. But there is no other option because self-love is the only key to happiness.

In other words, you are just as entitled to be happy as the next man and it isn't something you need to earn. Once you get rid of that inner bully, who has been making your life a misery for far too long, you will discover it is possible to be imperfect yet still lovable.

Do remember to keep your ego in check, though. Self-love isn't an excuse to be arrogant but a ticket to balance and harmony. By all means, believe in your capabilities and be proud of your positive qualities, but stay away from letting your ego take over the show. There is nothing worse than an overbearing guy who is full of himself and that's not what you should be aiming for.

Being quietly confident and modest says much more about your inner strength than any chest beating. You don't need to prove anything to anyone and when you feel good about who you are, that will speak for itself.

Your future begins now so don't let the past stop you. It's your time to become the man you always wanted to be and I am certain you will be a great success!

Highlights

- **There has never been a better time to be a man and escape the old-fashioned gender roles.**
- **Masculinity and maleness don't have to define who you are as a man.**
- **By appraising the personal beliefs you have about yourself, you can begin to see yourself more positively.**
- **Self-love is a habit you should incorporate into everyday life.**
- **Get into the habit of paying attention to your physical, mental, emotional, and spiritual needs.**
- **The habit of self-assessment will inspire and motivate you to seek greater self-love.**
- **The pursuit of happiness is a human right that everyone deserves to experience.**

9
A LOVE LETTER TO YOURSELF

"If you're searching for that one person that will change your life, take a look in the mirror." – **Roman Price**

In today's world of instant texting, emails, and emojis, writing a personal letter might sound ridiculous. Why bother doing that when you can just send a quick message on Viber, WhatsApp or Instagram?

If you belong to the generation that has never written a real letter before, I get your point. You might be able to stretch to a cute GIF or a sticky note, but that's about it, right? You older gents will recall the art of writing but could be a bit rusty and probably haven't written a proper letter for several years. Apart from that, the last thing on a man's mind would be to pick up a pen and start writing a love letter to himself – that's a woman thing, isn't it?

Despite what you might think, writing a love letter to yourself has become a popular trend, as well as the use of life journals and workbooks to help people nurture more self-awareness, and it's not only for women.

Everyone can benefit from the practice because it gives you the chance to reflect on where you are in life and to get in touch with your inner emotions. Let's face it – you aren't likely to get a love letter from anyone else in this digital age, but the power of the written word is still as strong as it ever was.

Add some self-love to that and you can begin to get closer to yourself, increase your self-awareness and to appreciate the person you are.

That's a weird idea!

Despite how weird it might sound to write a love letter to yourself, I suggest you give it a shot – what have you got to lose? While you may find it relatively easy to express your feelings about others, you probably don't spend any time expressing self-love and you should.

Introspective writing, as it is sometimes called, is an intimate, private activity that has multiple benefits. It's the ultimate self-care strategy for when you have forgotten to look after yourself or are feeling unhappy with your life.

- It reduces anxiety and stress.
- It reminds you that you need love and attention as much as anyone.
- It helps you feel loved.
- It boosts your self-esteem and self-regard.
- It helps you feel more confident and empowered.
- It's a safe space to express yourself without fear of judgment.
- It gives you a chance to communicate your deepest thoughts and emotions.
- It can help you to overcome mental health issues like anxiety or depression.
- It gives you something tangible to hold onto when you need encouragement and motivation.

Not so long ago, it was very common for people to keep diaries, where they would note their thoughts and feelings on a daily basis.

More recently, prompted journals have become fashionable, in which you are asked to regularly write about certain aspects of your life to improve your well-being.

A love letter to yourself can have the same effect, although you don't need to do it every day. It can be a one-off thing that you keep and look back on a month, a year, or ten years later. It's up to you how often you write one but you won't know how useful it is until you actually try it first.

How to write a love letter to yourself

Find what works for you

If you don't like the idea of writing on paper, you could use the notes app on your smartphone or create a document on your laptop. While real writing with pen and paper is better because it engages both your motor skills and senses, tapping it out on a keyboard is ok if that is what you feel most comfortable with.

Find a quiet time and space

Instead of scribbling something down in a hurry, dedicate a specific time when you know you won't be disturbed and haven't got any other plans.

Allow yourself about thirty minutes to an hour for your writing session and if you get stuck, take a five-minute break before continuing.

Find a comfy spot where you feel relaxed enough to write and get into the mood with some ambient background music and a nice cup of tea or coffee.

Write in the third person

That means writing to yourself as if you were writing to someone else, beginning with 'Dear ....' (add your name). This is a very effective way to help you feel calm and distance yourself from any intense emotions that may arise or feelings of overwhelm.

Imagine you are writing to someone you truly love and it should make it easier for you to get going.

Choose your approach

There are several different ways to write your love letter and you can choose the one that resonates with you the most.

You could simply begin without planning what to write and see what comes out, or you could follow prompts similar to the self-love declarations I asked you to complete in the previous chapter. Use sentences like:

One thing I love about you is that you ......

I admire you for your......

Another way to approach it is to write a letter to your past, present, or future self.

You might tap into emotions that have been buried for a long time or gain insights into the way you are feeling presently, as well as realize what you really want in your life.

It isn't always easy to delve into the past so if you feel uncomfortable doing so, there is no need to force yourself.

For now, focus on the present moment and write about how you are feeling as you write your very first letter.

What to write

The whole idea of writing a love letter to yourself is to express unconditional love for the person you are. It's not a confession of how badly you have behaved, or how useless you are. It isn't a self-critique or a chance to beat yourself up. It's an opportunity to practice pure self-love, no strings attached.

In your letter, you can:

- mention how you feel about yourself
- include your strengths and weaknesses
- talk about what you love most about yourself
- note down how you think you make others feel
- praise yourself for your achievements

- forgive yourself for past mistakes
- comfort your inner child
- tell yourself how wonderful you are

Below, you will find some useful prompts to help you get started:

I love how you… (*set boundaries, are kind to others, look after your health, work hard, are great company, are loyal…*)

I love that you are passionate about… (*your job, your family, animals, mountain climbing, the environment, cooking…*)

I'm so proud of you for… (*being a great friend, getting a promotion, reaching your goals, stopping smoking, passing your driving test…*)

You deserve to be… (*happy, healthy, content, successful, rewarded, admired…*)

Can you think of any more prompts that will express your love for yourself?

A sample love letter

Below is an example of a letter I wrote to myself that you can use for inspiration. Remember that you can write whatever you like in your love letter as it should reflect your individuality and uniqueness. It might look something like this:

Dear Rebecca,

It's been a long time since we talked and I wanted to tell you that you mean more to me than anything else in the world.

Maybe I don't tell you how much I love you as often as I should, which is why I am writing this letter to you now.

We've been through some tough times together, but you were always there for me, as I have been here for you. Nothing could make us lose that special connection and I hope it continues to grow with each day that passes. Even though we haven't been in touch as much as I would have liked recently, never doubt my love for you, which is as deep as the ocean.

I love you for many reasons and admire how beautiful, caring, and strong you are. The truth is, you are the one I look up to – you are my role model – my superhero.

I love the way you care so much for your family and are always there for them when they need you.

I love how you will go out of your way to help a friend in need.

I love how you are so passionate about your work and want to share that passion with those around you.

I love your positivity and how you never let problems get you down or stop you from trying to be your very best.

I love your quirky sense of humor and the way you make people laugh.

I love how brave you are, even when you might not be feeling that courageous on the inside.

I love your smile.

You are very special to me and I want you to always remember that.

I promise to respect, honor, and cherish you forever more.

All my love,

Me

A letter to your future self

You might enjoy writing a letter to your future self, which you can promise to open again in a year's time, five years from now, or even decades later. The good thing about doing this kind of letter is that it allows you to reflect on how you see yourself in the future and what you would like to achieve.

It also gives your future self the chance to see what changes you have gone through in your life when you read it, and that can be quite insightful.

In the letter, talk about the hopes and dreams for the man you want to become. What will he be doing? Where will he be? Will he have a family? Is he successful in his career? What ideals does he live by? What goals has he achieved?

When you read the letter again, as your future self, in a year or several years from now, you might find that some of your goals and ideals have changed. It could be that you traded them for better ones and have matured into someone to be truly proud of.

You might look back at your younger self and recall how you felt when you wrote that letter, and thank yourself for doing so.

If you have not lived up to your own expectations and wandered from the path, the letter may even bring you back to your core values and help you revive old dreams and goals.

It can prompt you to reassess where you are, what you did wrong, and inspire you to become the man you always wanted to be. It's never too late for that to happen if you really wish for it.

Writing a love letter to yourself can be healing, therapeutic, and rewarding. It allows you to express your feelings and thoughts without fear of criticism and can help you to nurture greater self-love. That is definitely something worth doing so don't hold back – love yourself deeply and give yourself a huge big man hug.

Now, doesn't that feel great?

Highlights

- **Writing a love letter to yourself is the ultimate self-care activity.**
- **It has many benefits, like reducing anxiety and raising your self-esteem.**
- **Unlike journals that require regular writing, you only need to do it once.**
- **You can write your love letter on your smartphone or laptop if you prefer.**
- **It's an opportunity to dedicate some time for self-reflection without judgment.**

- **You can write freestyle or follow prompts to express how you feel.**
- **You can write to your future self about your dreams, goals, and expectations.**
- **It's an opportunity to practice pure, unconditional self-love.**

AFTERWORD

Everyone needs love. It's a universal human right and without it, life can be miserable. Our deep-rooted instinct to survive means that we search for love from the day we are born. We need to be cared for, nurtured, and loved if we are to grow into healthy, well-balanced adults.

Some of us get off to a bad start and our needs are not met, or life brings us setbacks that make us feel unworthy of being loved. By the time we reach adulthood, we are also carrying a lot of preconceived ideas around with us about what it means to be a man.

Cutting through all of that noise and getting in touch with our authentic selves isn't easy. Society exerts an incredible amount of pressure on us about how to behave, think, and feel. Gender stereotypes can restrict our self-expression and keep us locked in a role that doesn't really define us.

It takes a lot of inner strength and determination to stand up and say, "I'm not going along with this anymore."

No one wants to go against the norm and risk being ridiculed for behaving in a way that defies stereotypes.. When men are supposed to be tough, mean, aggressive, uncaring, and dominant, appearing to be otherwise can incite mockery and insult.

The irony is, that some of the most influential male leaders in history were compassionate men who believed in atypical masculine traits, such as non-violence and peaceful dialogue. Think of Mahatma Gandhi, Martin Luther King, Buddha, and Jesus himself, and you will see what I mean.

In our changing world, many young men are confused about their identity, not knowing how to react, respond, and behave. This has led to a mental health crisis but unfortunately, many of them feel unable to reach out for help and suffer in silence. Feelings of self-loathing, insecurity, and low self-esteem are aggravated by ideas of toxic masculinity, leaving many men feeling unlovable and unable to express themselves.

I hope that, after reading this book, you will feel bold enough to challenge the low opinion you may have had of yourself and find greater happiness in your life. By focusing on self-love, I have given you the key to unlock the door that is imprisoning you. All you need to do is turn it and set yourself free.

We talked about how boys learn to become men and why the way you were brought up doesn't have to define you as a person. You will recall how being vulnerable is a strength, not a weakness, and how self-love can liberate you from negative ideas about expressing your emotions.

We also looked at what self-love means in practice and I gave you some tools to help you assess how much it is lacking in your life and practical strategies to begin experiencing it. You will also have read about the long-lasting effects of trauma and why some men hurt others. I hope you will have gained some insights into why your behavior and perceptions need to change and have found my suggestions useful.

Throughout this book, the message has been focused on loving yourself, which then allows you to love others more and establish healthier relationships. Everyone has a different story, but if you can raise your levels of self-awareness and understand your actions more, the greater control you will have over your own life and the lives of those around you.

If you suffer from low self-esteem, you will have found some useful activities in the book to evaluate where that is coming from, as well as learn how to overcome it. Knowing more about what most women find attractive in men will also hopefully help you to focus on cultivating those qualities instead of worrying excessively about your appearance.

You will also have found many suggestions on how to bolster your self-worth and emotional well-being by helping others, which is an act of self-love itself.

Finally, it is my sincere wish that you begin to incorporate more self-love habits into your daily life and start to nourish your physical, emotional, mental, and spiritual well-being. From having a good night's sleep to writing yourself a love letter, each small act can help you to feel empowered.

Good luck on your journey and remember: you deserve to be loved for who you are – a kind, caring, strong, passionate man.

Be fearless, be bold, and love yourself deeply. There is no greater gift you can give yourself in life!

Could I ask you a favour?. would you spare 2 minutes to write an honest review for this book from wherever you bought it. Reviews mean such a lot to me. Thanks in advance.

Rebecca x

Other Books By Rebecca Collins

Love Yourself Deeply

How To Make Friends Easily

Love Yourself Deeply & How To Make Friends Easily 2 in 1 Book

The Art Of Manifesting Money

Help!, I'm a Teenager

Positive Life Skills For Teens

SOURCES

Mental Health Foundation UK, 1 October 2021

https://www.apa.org/monitor/2015/12/numbers

Pediatrics (2014) 134 (6): e1603–e1610. https://doi.org/10.1542/peds.2013-4289

Front. Psychol., 24 September 2013 Sec. Developmental Psychology

https://doi.org/10.3389/fpsyg.2013.00670

Grayson P., The Descent of Man, Penguin Books (2017)

https://youtu.be/c77HKCYq9XE

https://www.sciencedirect.com/science/article/pii/S0022399913003036?casa_token=Ov2aCtQs6xYAAAAA:t_Jp4t51cdE63wouedkRKLnuPPfe2hEMNxJpJ2xHAwwBzDa5qKNwWog_UqZr2oHV50gpq2g-gQ

https://www.sciencedirect.com/science/article/abs/pii/S0010440X18300555

https://www.ons.gov.uk/peoplepopulationandcommunity/crimeandjustice/articles/homicideinenglandandwales/yearendingmarch2021

https://wwwdev.cdc.gov/violenceprevention/datasources/nisvs/index.html

Feder, J., Levant, R. F., & Dean, J. (2010). Boys and violence: A gender-informed analysis. Psychology of Violence, 1(S), 3–12. https://doi.org/10.1037/2152-0828.1.S.3

Baugher, A. R., & Gazmararian, J. A. (2015). Masculine gender role stress and violence: A literature review and future directions. Aggression and Violent Behavior, 24, 107–112. https://doi.org/10.1016/j.avb.2015.04.002

Lundy, D. E., Tan, J., & Cunningham, M. R. (1998). Heterosexual romantic preferences: The importance of humour and physical attractiveness for different types of relationships. Personal Relationships, 5, 311–325.

https://www.sciencedirect.com/science/article/abs/pii/S0191886915001336

http://www.sirc.org/publik/smell_attract.html

Renninger, LeeAnn et al. "Getting that female glance: Patterns and consequences of male nonverbal behavior in courtship contexts." *Evolution and Human Behavior* 25 (2004): 416-431.

https://www.sciencedirect.com/science/article/abs/pii/S0191886908001748?via%3Dihub#!

https://pubmed.ncbi.nlm.nih.gov/27100366/

https://academic.oup.com/gerontologist/article/54/5/830/627130

Dr. Ted Zeff, *Raise an Emotionally Healthy Boy*: Save Your Son From the Violent Boy Culture, Prana Publishing, 2013

https://psychologydictionary.org/maleness/

https://happinessday.org/wp-content/uploads/2015/11/UN66281.pdf

NOTES

INTRODUCTION

1. Mental Health Foundation UK, **1 October 2021**
2. https://www.apa.org/monitor/2015/12/numbers

2. FROM BOYS TO MEN

1. *Pediatrics* (2014) 134 (6): e1603–e1610. https://doi.org/10.1542/peds.2013-4289
2. Front. Psychol., 24 September 2013 Sec. Developmental Psychology https://doi.org/10.3389/fpsyg.2013.00670
3. Grayson P., The Descent of Man, Penguin Books 2017

3. BIG BOYS DO CRY

1. https://www.sciencedirect.com/science/article/pii/S0022399913003036?casa_token=Ov2aCtQs6xYAAAAA:t_Jp4t51cdE63wouedkRKLnuPPfe2hEMNxJpJ2x-HAwwBzDa5qKNwWog_UqZr20HV50gpq2g-gQ
2. https://www.sciencedirect.com/science/article/abs/pii/S0010440X18300555

4. MEN WHO HURT OTHERS ARE OFTEN HURT THEMSELVES

1. https://www.ons.gov.uk/peoplepopulationandcommunity/crimeandjustice/articles/homicideinenglandandwales/yearendingmarch2021
2. National Intimate Partner and Sexual Violence Survey
3. Feder, J., Levant, R. F., & Dean, J. (2010). Boys and violence: A gender-informed analysis. Psychology of Violence, 1(S), 3–12. https://doi.org/10.1037/2152-0828.1.S.3
4. Baugher, A. R., & Gazmararian, J. A. (2015). Masculine gender role stress and violence: A literature review and future directions. Aggression and Violent Behavior, 24, 107–112. https://doi.org/10.1016/j.avb.2015.04.002

6. THE 7 TOP TURN ONS IN MEN

1. Lundy, D. E., Tan, J., & Cunningham, M. R. (1998). Heterosexual romantic preferences: The importance of humour and physical attractiveness for different types of relationships. Personal Relationships, 5, 311–325.
2. https://www.sciencedirect.com/science/article/abs/pii/S0191886915001336
3. http://www.sirc.org/publik/smell_attract.html

4. Renninger, LeeAnn et al. "Getting that female glance: Patterns and consequences of male nonverbal behavior in courtship contexts." *Evolution and Human Behavior* 25 (2004): 416-431.
5. https://www.sciencedirect.com/science/article/abs/pii/S0191886908001748?via%3Dihub#!

7. ARE YOU HELPING OR HURTING OTHERS?

1. https://pubmed.ncbi.nlm.nih.gov/27100366/
2. https://academic.oup.com/gerontologist/article/54/5/830/627130

8. IT'S TIME TO PUT IT ALL INTO PRACTICE

1. https://psychologydictionary.org/maleness/
2. https://happinessday.org/wp-content/uploads/2015/11/UN66281.pdf

www.ingramcontent.com/pod-product-compliance
Lightning Source LLC
Chambersburg PA
CBHW041145110526
44590CB00027B/4130